HAVING YOUR
BABY WITH A
NURSE-MIDWIFE

HAVING YOUR BABY WITH A NURSE-MIDWIFE

Everything You Need to Know to Make an Informed Decision

The American College of Nurse-Midwives

and Sandra Jacobs

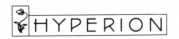

NEW YORK

618.2
Jac

This book is intended to give basic information about the role of nurse-midwifery in childbearing and about choosing a midwife. The information contained in this book is not intended to be and should not be construed as medical advice, or as a substitute for regular prenatal and other medical consultation. If you have a question about your own pregnancy, labor, and delivery, or about any other medical or physical condition, consult your nurse-midwife, doctor, or health-care organization to receive specific advice.

Library of Congress Cataloging-in-Publication Data
Jacobs, Sandra.
Having your baby with a nurse-midwife : everything you need to know to make an informed decision / by the American College of Nurse-Midwives and Sandra Jacobs.—1st ed.
p.   cm.
Includes bibliographical references.
ISBN 1-56282-860-6
1. Midwives.   2. Pregnancy.   3. Childbirth.   I. American College of Nurse-Midwives.   II. Title.
RG950.J33   1993
618.2'0233—dc20   92-36373
CIP

First Edition
10   9   8   7   6   5   4   3   2   1

Acknowledgments

TRUE MIDWIFE to this book is Howard Morhaim who had the good sense to suggest the project and the perseverance to see it through. The wisdom and support of Dr. Joyce Thompson, president of the American College of Nurse-Midwives, made the book possible.

Three guardian angels from the American College of Nurse-Midwives tirelessly read drafts and made suggestions: Sister Jeanne Meurer, CNM; Sister Angela Murdaugh, CNM, and Lisa Summers, CNM. Special thanks to Mary Hammond-Tooke, CNM, for assistance on the home birth chapter and to Lisa Paine, CNM for guidance on new research.

Fort Lauderdale friends offered sharp eyes, insight and encouragement: Barbara Walsh, Deborah Work, Ardy and Suzy Friedberg, and especially Ellen Forman.

Susan Schwartz provided valuable guidance in shaping initial chapters. Vicki DiStasio's editing and enthusiasm kept me and the project on track.

Those most responsible for this book, however, are the mothers, families and nurse-midwives who opened their lives and told their stories. To them, this book is dedicated.

Contents

1.

WHAT IS A NURSE-MIDWIFE?

NANCY JUST COULD not push anymore. She knew the baby was almost there, but suddenly overwhelmed by panic, she felt unable to cope with those final contractions.

Then she heard a calm, familiar voice.

"It's really hard, I know," Dianne, her nurse-midwife said. "But you can do it."

With the next contraction, Nancy gave one more push. Then one more. Her husband Donald moved to the foot of the hospital bed. "It's beautiful," he gasped as the crown of their baby's head pushed its way into the world.

Nancy shut her eyes and focused on her nurse-midwife's voice.

"Don't push now, just breathe," said Dianne, as she eased out the baby's head. Next came a stubborn shoulder. "Now push," Dianne said. "Slow, slow."

Then Donald took over. With the final push, the father grasped his own baby—a daughter!—and placed her on Nancy's belly. He covered the squirming infant with a warm receiving blanket as Nancy moaned and laughed with relief. With hugs and caresses, the parents welcomed 8-pound, 3-ounce Rebecca.

How different it had been when their first daughter was born. They had been shuttled from one hospital room to the next, Nancy groggy from medication and hooked up to an intravenous line and electronic monitoring equipment. In the delivery room, she was scolded when she instinctively reached down to touch her baby. Donald was not allowed to hold the newborn until the child was bathed and swaddled.

With this second baby, their hospital room felt festive. In labor, Nancy padded around in her flowered kimono as she played her favorite Bette Midler and Barbra Streisand tapes. Because Dianne encouraged her to sip juice and water, she needed no intravenous lines. She did not even think about pain medication; until those final few minutes, the contractions seemed manageable. When the pains came closer together, Nancy sat in the rocking chair, while Dianne breathed with her and coached her through each one.

Nancy was wide awake when Rebecca was born. She nursed the baby immediately. Within minutes, three-year-old Rachel joined her family, climbing onto the bed for a hug from her mother and a wide-eyed hello to her baby sister.

Dianne stayed with them, making sure mother and baby were all right. Nancy loved how Rebecca never had to leave her sight. She felt connected to her baby, and proud of the calm, joyful and healthy birth. She had felt that same calm and confidence throughout pregnancy with her nurse-midwives Dianne and Sharron. As childbirth experts, they performed checkups and provided a never-ending stream of advice, encouragement and information, including Nancy and Donald in all decisions. Nancy liked that feeling of control. As a woman and mother, she felt responsible for the life growing inside her and liked being part of her baby's care from the very start.

By the time of that second pregnancy, Nancy was a successful lawyer who had tasted all sorts of achievements in her thirty-three years. But none was as sweet as the birth of Rebecca.

"This was different," she said. "I felt a real sense of accomplishment, as a woman. I *gave birth* to this child. And she and I are very close."

A joyful and healthy start is what having a baby with a nurse-midwife is all about. Childbearing is a normal part of life and need not be treated as an illness. But a pregnant woman does need professional guidance and emotional support. Nurse-midwives know the strength of women and the natural beauty of childbirth. With the guidance, assistance and understanding of a nurse-midwife, pregnancy and birth can be made even healthier and more joyful.

A certified nurse-midwife is a registered nurse who has additional education in midwifery—the care of healthy, pregnant women and newborns. By education and experience, a nurse-midwife is qualified to be the main caregiver throughout pregnancy and childbirth for healthy women, and to provide gynecological and family planning care throughout a woman's childbearing years. Each year, more than a hundred thousand women in the United States give birth to their babies with the help of nurse-midwives. The numbers continue to grow as word spreads that having a baby with a nurse-midwife is a satisfying experience.

If you are having your baby with a nurse-midwife, she

is the person you see during prenatal visits. She monitors your health, makes sure the fetus is growing properly and answers your questions. She remains by your side during labor, checking the fetus, helping you cope with contractions, and finally assisting you in delivering your baby. A doctor need not be present for prenatal visits, labor, or delivery with a nurse-midwife, but one is available if needed.

The nurse-midwife approach to childbirth is "low tech," based on the philosophy that birth proceeds well on its own when allowed to follow nature's fine-tuned engineering. Nurse-midwifery does not reject the use of medical technology such as medication, sonograms, electronic fetal monitoring, if the situation calls for it. But if birth is progressing well on its own, none of these procedures are used automatically.

The four thousand nurse-midwives in the United States can be found working in all fifty states, with the largest concentration in California, followed by New York, Florida, Pennsylvania, Illinois, Massachusetts, and Texas. They work in private practices, universities, hospitals, health maintenance organizations (HMOs), birth centers, and public clinics. In addition to childbirth-related care, nurse-midwives provide regular gynecological services throughout a woman's life, including yearly pelvic exams, breast exams, and pap smears, preconception care and family planning. In thirty-three states and the District of Columbia, nurse-midwives can write prescriptions. Nurse-midwives do not perform cesarean sections. They do not perform abortions. Insurance companies and Medicaid cover nurse-midwife care in most states.

Many people envision birth at home when they hear the word "midwife." But the vast majority of nurse-midwives work in hospitals—about 85 percent. Another 11 percent work in birth centers, and the remaining 4 percent attend home births. Regardless of the setting, nurse-midwives approach birth as an event that belongs to a family, not a medical system. Fathers, siblings, grandparents, and friends can be included in the celebration of a new life. Parents are allowed, indeed expected, to take part in all decisions relating to the birth of their child.

EDUCATION

A nurse-midwife is a registered nurse who typically has worked in maternity or public health nursing before entering nurse-midwifery school. In 1992, there were thirty-one educational programs accredited by the American College of Nurse-Midwives (ACNM) at such prestigious universities as Yale, Emory, Columbia, and the University of California at San Francisco and at San Diego. In these nurse-midwifery schools, students spend eighteen months to two years learning clinical midwifery skills, advanced obstetrics/gynecology for normal women, newborn care, and family planning. Most of the programs lead to master's degrees. Others are certificate programs or precertification programs for midwives who trained outside the U.S. or have been out of practice for a while. To become certified, a nurse-midwifery school graduate must pass the rigorous exam of the ACNM Certification Council, Inc., and then meet state requirements to practice.

Nurse-midwives are often confused with other types of midwives, who may have less formal education and primarily do home births. These midwives generally are not nurses. Some attend midwife training programs and most serve an apprenticeship with another midwife. Some states license these non-nurse midwives; in others they work "underground." These midwives extend from a tradition of women helping women in childbirth from the early New England midwives who played a crucial role in the social fabric of their communities to the "granny mid-wives" who still work in pockets of the rural south. But the continued use of midwives who are not certified nurse-midwives has been controversial. These midwives will be discussed further in chapters on home birth and the politics of midwifery. Throughout this book, however, the terms nurse-midwife, CNM (certified nurse-midwife), and midwife all refer to nurse-midwives who have been certified by the American College of Nurse-Midwives or the ACNM Certification Council, Inc.

MOTIVATION

Nurse-midwives in the U.S. come to their profession from a wide variety of backgrounds, although most have experience as labor and delivery nurses before attending nurse-midwifery school. They turn to midwifery because they want to be involved in the whole triumph of a pregnancy and birth, not just a small slice, and they want more responsibility than they had as nurses. Some become interested when they have a child of their own, and feel the lack of a personal dimension. Most nurse-midwives choose their profession in order to play a role in improving women's health care and to bring out the best of the childbirth experience. All relish nurse-midwifery's emphasis on the joyful aspects of good health and women's special strengths—with a tangible result nestled in a mother's arms.

Despite the repeated use of "she" when referring to a nurse-midwife, there are in fact male nurse-midwives in the U.S., although they make up less than 1 percent of the total. Most of them received their education and early experience in the military. Throughout this book, however, nurse-midwives will be described in the female gender. This is only in deference to the majority, and certainly is not intended to be a slight or to exclude male nurse-midwives, who share the same dedication and devotion to the women they care for as their female colleagues.

Regardless of why they became nurse-midwives, nearly all see their profession as a calling, something they enjoy and were meant to do. Leslie Stewart, a nurse-midwife who does home births in Los Angeles, said many nurse-midwives seem destined for their work. When she began the obstetrical portion of nursing school, she found no need to study; it seemed to come naturally, by instinct. When she graduated from nurse-midwifery school, her mother congratulated her on her persistence.

"I don't remember it, but my mother says that when I was five years old, I told her, 'I'm gonna born the babies,' " Leslie said. "How could I have known that? I think with the best midwives, it's inborn."

Nurse-midwifery is striving to maintain the spiritual dimension that grows from the wonder of birth, in the face of an increasingly technological world. The history of women helping women is part of their profession, even in its most modern form. Daily, nurse-midwives meet the challenge of combining that caring legacy with modern technology to help make birth safer and more satisfying than ever.

CHILDBIRTH EXPERTS

Certified nurse-midwives are fully educated and qualified to be the primary caregivers for normal pregnancy and birth, and they work in affiliation with a physician should complications develop. That doctor, generally an obstetrician/gynecologist, is available for consultation and/or referral if needed at any time during the pregnancy. If a medical complication arises in labor, the physician takes over the care.

The arrangement between doctors and nurse-midwives has been set forth in a series of joint statements, beginning in 1971, between the American College of Nurse-Midwives and the American College of Obstetricians and Gynecologists. The two professional groups have agreed that a nurse-midwife may be responsible for the complete care of maternity patients who have no complications, provided that the nurse-midwife is part of a team that includes an obstetrician. Both professional groups recommend that nurse-midwives and the doctors who work with them define their roles in written agreements that make clear everything from money matters to the medical conditions for which the doctor will be consulted.

About one in six pregnant women require a doctor's attention for conditions that existed before pregnancy or for complications that develop during pregnancy and labor. The other five women experience the normal childbirth that is the expertise of nurse-midwives. A normal pregnancy means the mother remains healthy—normal blood pressure, normal metabolism, no infections—and the placenta and fetus develop properly. During labor, normal means that the heart-rate of mother and child remain in a certain range and labor progresses requiring little medical intervention. Nurse-midwives' eyes and hands are so well-attuned to what is normal in pregnancy and labor that they are quick to recognize any deviations.

Nurse-midwife policy is to consult with a doctor as soon as a pregnancy or labor steers toward any condition that is considered medically dangerous. Whether the problem is apparent during the first prenatal visit or does not arise until the final hour of labor, a nurse-midwife is taught to call in a doctor as soon as the woman's condition strays outside the boundaries of a nurse-midwife's expertise. The mother may be referred to the consulting doctor for medical care, or the physician and nurse-mid-wife may co-manage care, depending on the complication.

Over the years, nurse-midwives have maintained a superb record of safety. Research shows that pregnancy, labor, and delivery for a healthy woman is as safe with a nurse-midwife as with a physician. And women in the care of nurse-midwives are less likely to have cesarean sections, forceps births, and episiotomies. While medical experts have begun to question the high U.S. rate of cesarean birth and the routine use of invasive procedures in childbirth, government reports have called for an increased use of nurse-midwives as a safe way to improve maternity care. (See Chapter 7.)

Nurse-midwives screen women rigorously and accept only women whose good health prior to pregnancy makes them low-risk for developing complications. High-risk women, those who have more potential for problems during pregnancy because of medical conditions such as heart disease or diabetes, belong in the care of a doctor.

Nurse-midwives have been particularly successful in improving birth results among teenagers and women who have low incomes. For some, social or economic situations can add stress to pregnancy. Nurse-midwives help identify the unhealthy factors and then work to minimize the risks—seeing that a woman gets food assistance if she qualifies financially, encouraging her to alter abusive situations, explaining how drugs, alcohol, and tobacco can harm a fetus, and how good nutrition helps. Nurse-midwives have demonstrated great success in working with women to prevent psychological or social risk factors from causing medical or obstetrical complications during pregnancy or labor. In some settings, particularly public clinics, nurse-midwives may share with doctors the care of women who have some high-risk factors. Women who do not purposely choose nurse-midwives, but encounter them at their clinic or hospital, come away feeling there is something different about having a baby with a nurse-midwife—a little extra love and attention.

Obstetrician/gynecologists have years of specialized training and experience with the medical and obstetrical complications that may arise in pregnancy and childbirth and in the other pathologies of female reproduction. Much of that expertise, however, is not needed for a healthy pregnant woman. The professional challenge for obstetricians is to treat successfully those women and babies who are threatened by illness or abnormality; that is the goal for which they spend years preparing and the one that brings them the most satisfaction. When nurse-midwives attend to healthy pregnant women, doctors are free to spend time on the illnesses they are trained to cure.

A CELEBRITY'S VIEW, A WOMAN'S CHOICE

Actress Cybill Shepherd drew from her own experience when she called nurse-midwives "absolutely the best choice for women."

"There's no way a doctor can ever give a woman during pregnancy or labor what a nurse-midwife can give," she said. "Doctors are trained for abnormalities in birth. Nurse-midwives are the artists of normal birth."

When Cybill became pregnant with Clementine in the late 1970s, she found a doctor she liked very much at the University of Tennessee in her hometown of Memphis. He referred her to a birth class taught by nurse-midwives. Cybill liked the nurse-midwives and their approach. As she read about childbirth, she drew some conclusions: if a woman was surrounded by caregivers of her own choosing, people she knew well and trusted, mother and baby would fare best. She asked her doctor the likelihood of his being there for the birth. His answer: 90 percent. If she switched to the nurse-midwives, she asked, how likely would one be with her? The answer: 100 percent.

"So right there was the difference," she said. "One of these people who you were so close to, who you saw all through pregnancy, could be with you for the birth. You have more of a chance to build trust."

With her doctor's agreement, Cybill switched to the nurse-midwives. She liked their openness and emphasis on education; she felt well prepared.

"As you learn about what is going to happen to you in birth, or the many different possibilities that can happen, your fear quotient goes down. As you overcome that fear, your chance of discomfort and pain is lessened."

Cybill does not hide the fact that her thirty-one-hour labor was painful, but the nurse-midwives made an immeasurable difference. "I'm sure I would have had a cesarean had I not been with nurse-midwives," she said. "They worked with me so carefully."

After thirty hours, she was exhausted. The nurse-midwives gave her a regional anesthetic so the pain would not sap her strength. As it wore off, she asked for more. It would be Cybill's choice whether to receive more anesthesia, the nurse-midwife explained, but she made clear one possible outcome: it might inhibit Cybill from pushing effectively, making a forceps birth more likely. Between contractions, Cybill asked how close she was to giving birth. The midwife looked at the clock, then 6:20 p.m., and said Cybill would have her baby by seven. Cybill chose to let the anesthesia wear off.

"I trusted her, and I believed in her," Cybill said. "I don't think anybody except the nurse-midwife who had been with me—not just for labor, but for the whole pregnancy, too—could make me feel that much trust. She had

been with me through all the pain and difficulty, breathing with me, helping me, supporting me. So when she
said, 'You can do it,' I believed her."

It was that "leap of faith," Cybill said, that gave her
the strength to deliver her baby. Clementine, 8½ pounds,
was born at 6:59. Cybill did not need an episiotomy, and
for that she credits the skill of her nurse-midwife.

> She stood right there with me and said, "Okay, a little
> push, a little bigger, now a little less push." We managed,
> through communication, to orchestrate the very gentle
> birth of that child. It never could have happened without
> a midwife who knew that art.
>
> The thing about birth is that you know you're going to
> lose control. There is that point you want to give up. It's
> usually right before you start to push the baby out, and
> they call it "transition." You need all the help you can
> get. To not have a nurse-midwife is to go without a cru-
> cial kind of help. When you get down to it, everyone
> except the mother is a birth attendant. Nobody is going
> to go through labor but you; no one else is going to push
> that baby out. So it's good to have with you someone
> you know well, who will be there the whole time.
>
> Birth is such a powerful thing. You confront the most
> primitive thing, the incredible force of nature, and you
> need the support of women. You need that enormous
> support. For pregnancy, birth control, anything, I saw
> the first place to go is nurse-midwives.

After Clementine's birth, Cybill continued routine care
with nurse-midwives.

HEALTHY BODY AND SOUL

Nurse-midwives begin with the premise that pregnancy
is a normal condition until proven otherwise. They watch

for key health indicators that might prove otherwise—
abnormally high blood pressure or slow growth of the
fetus, for instance. But they also regard other aspects of
your well-being. They approach pregnancy holistically,
as an experience that affects you emotionally as well as
physically. Even when pregnancy is healthy and normal,
it can bring with it a host of physical discomforts, for
which nurse-midwives have all sorts of remedies, some
medical, others simply homespun good sense. Because
nurse-midwives also are attuned to the emotional and
psychological aspects of birth, they address a wide spectrum of needs. Fear of labor, anxiety about being a parent, concern about stretch marks, may be very real issues
for you, and your nurse-midwife helps you address them.

Often a nurse-midwife takes her cues from you, gaug-
ing the kind of personal support that you as an individual
need. You know your own body better than anyone else
does. A nurse-midwife encourages you to listen to your
body, and she listens to you. Throughout the pregnancy,
her goal is to help you maintain good health, emotionally
and physically, so that you feel confident and positive about
the pregnancy.

Pregnancy is demanding, physically and emotionally,
no matter how healthy you are. Your feet may ache, your
body may appear all wrong to you, and you may go from
nausea to heartburn. If you respond by thinking that these
things necessarily mean you are ill, you may begin to regard childbirth as a process in which you give up responsibility for yourself. A nurse-midwife helps you cope with
normal ailments while preserving the image of yourself
as a healthy and responsible adult. Pregnancy need not
diminish a woman; rather, it can be an empowering experience. A nurse-midwife can help you nurture, in childbirth, the strength that grows from feeling responsible
and in control.

Your nurse-midwife is your partner in bringing you

closer and closer to delivering a healthy baby, and she can help you to have the kind of experience you want. But as in any partnership, each participant is expected to play an active role. A nurse-midwife may listen endlessly to your concerns and patiently answer question after question. She will explain to you your options, inform you of possible outcomes. But it is up to you as a parent to define your pregnancy. Ultimately, you make your own choices—from what you eat or drink during pregnancy to who will witness the birth.

Even a nurse-midwife's language reflects her notion of who is ultimately in charge when it comes to having a baby. Rarely will she say that *she* delivers babies. The mother, after all, is the one who feels the powerful contractions that propel a new life into the world. But the nurse-midwife, your partner throughout, is right there with you, to assist and guide you.

PREPARED CHILDBIRTH

Having a baby with a nurse-midwife is sometimes described as "natural childbirth," but the term "prepared childbirth" that has come to use in recent years is more accurate. Prepared childbirth means parents learn about the childbirth process by taking classes and reading about it. They learn enough to be involved in all aspects of the pregnancy and birth, from maintaining good health and nutrition habits to being included in all decisions about their care. The decision of how "natural" the birth will be is left up to the parents.

One of the most significant roles of a nurse-midwife is teaching—making you aware of what is happening during pregnancy and preparing you for labor. A health professional's explanation that he or she will take care of everything may be vaguely reassuring, but it does not prepare you to have a baby. Nurse-midwives make sure you have ample knowledge and realistic expectations. They do not tell you that birth is going to be easy; in fact it may be the most difficult thing you ever have done. It also may be the most rewarding.

Through nine months of prenatal care, women develop a trust with their nurse-midwives based on full disclosure, an open ear, two-way communication, and sound advice. This trust is one of a woman's greatest resources when labor begins.

TECHNOLOGY IN ITS PLACE

You may wonder: what if I want pain medication? And will a nurse-midwife allow a sonogram, or use electronic fetal monitoring? A common misconception about nurse-midwives is that they forgo all pain medication and technology, and that women in their care must ascribe to a "tough it out" mentality. That is rarely true. Certainly, it is possible to have a completely natural childbirth with a nurse-midwife, and most see that as the ideal. But many nurse-midwives also make available pain medication. Their professional standards also include using what medical science has to offer—when warranted.

When warranted is the key behind a nurse-midwife's use of medical intervention. A nurse-midwife does not believe that technology should be turned to simply because it is there; she prefers to use the least invasive measures to help a woman before turning to technological help that could also have side effects. For instance, if a woman's labor slows down, a nurse-midwife commonly encourages her to walk or to try different positions before resorting to labor-inducing drugs. Nurse-midwives know how to work patiently to ease the baby over the mother's perineum, rather than routinely make an episiotomy (a cut in the perineal tissue).

Nurse-midwife practice may include using a fetal monitor, a sonogram, or an episiotomy, if it will help a woman and if the potential benefits outweigh the risks. But along with the technology, they offer the strong dose of human contact that characterizes midwifery care.

WHAT MOTHERS SAY

• "They are the most down-to-earth, honest, human, caring people I've ever met," said Louise, a Los Angeles mother whose four children were born into the hands of nurse-midwives. Her first three children were born in a Denver birth center; her youngest was born with a nurse-midwife at home after the family moved to California. Louise found that the personal attention and reassurances of her nurse-midwives kept her confident, especially when the strains of pregnancy were taking a toll on her. Her nurse-midwives understood that pregnancy was not just a physical condition, but one that affected a woman's emotions and family life.

"You can talk to them about everything under the sun, whether it's sex or school or about how your other kids are driving you crazy," Louise said. "That understanding helps a woman feel good about herself. When you feel good about yourself, you're going to have a healthy baby.

"It's neat to have someone who cares so much. They spend time with you. They don't just walk in when you're ready and say, 'Push!' The miracle of life should be taken as something neat, not something yucky. If you concentrate on the baby coming out, it's wonderful."

• Sarah, during the course of her three pregnancies, saw a total of four or five nurse-midwives in a group practice in Palm Beach County, Florida. No matter which nurse-midwife was involved, she always felt it was someone who genuinely cared about her.

"When you enter a relationship with a nurse-midwife you end up with a friend," she said. "You get more than you bargain for."

The nurse-midwife with whom she felt the strongest bond was by her side during the hospital births of all three babies. Her experiences led her to conclude that nurse-midwives were an unusual breed of professionals.

"They have a real passion for what they're doing," she said. "They love what they're doing and it comes through. It's a special kind of devotion."

• Jane, a lawyer and first-time mother in New York, interviewed six obstetricians and three nurse-midwives and scoured books about childbirth during the first weeks of her pregnancy before she chose a nurse-midwife practice. She shopped for maternity care the same way she would for any other professional service, placing high priority on the professional's expertise for the particular task at hand. If she were evaluating a lawyer's services, she would ask: How many times have you done that business transaction? In her mind, a person's ability to do a job well is often based on experience.

"What I liked about the midwives is that they are baby delivery specialists," she said. "They know this stuff, they've seen lots of women who have delivered, had this type of pain, or had this type of itchiness. They know how to [help you] deal with it. Or they know you can't deal with it. You can't trade that kind of experience."

WHAT DOCTORS SAY

The practice of Dr. Paul Gaither, an obstetrician-gynecologist outside Boston, includes four doctors and six nurse-midwives. Gaither was pleased when the first two nurse-midwives came to him and his partner in the early 1980s, seeking to work with them. The doctors had been frustrated, feeling that their care of pregnant women was incomplete; they had neither time nor suitable background to teach women about pregnancy and offer the support a pregnant woman needs. The nurse-midwives had the time and inclination, during both pregnancy and labor.

"Physicians are taught to deal with pathology," Dr. Gaither said, "but don't know what the heck to do with well people. Nurse-midwives are intelligent, well-trained practitioners who can teach us a lot. . . . If patients ask I tell them I think it's the best of both worlds to have a CNM [Certified Nurse-Midwife] delivery. A doctor won't sit with you in labor. When you have a delivery with a doctor, a labor room nurse is the first line of defense. She'll call us if there is a problem. If there is a nurse-midwife, this is a much more highly trained person who will be quicker to pick up abnormality. We're in the background if a major complication occurs."

One woman who had her first baby in another physician's practice came to Dr. Gaither's practice for her second baby. After the first few months of alternating doctor and nurse-midwife visits she asked Dr. Gaither's advice on whom she should choose for the remainder of pregnancy and birth. His response: "You had a normal delivery last time, you are healthy, you probably will have a normal delivery again. So enjoy yourself with this one—go with the midwife."

Many physicians who work with nurse-midwives are happy to see their wives and daughters give birth with nurse-midwives—it means the pregnancy is normal and healthy. The wife of Dr. Irving Robinson, a New York City obstetrician who is consulting physician for a nurse-midwife practice, had both their sons with the nurse-midwifery practice.

"It was my wife's choice, I wanted her to be comfortable," Dr. Robinson said. "There's a lot of room for relaxation of the stringent rules and regulations of how we treat people. . . . The nurse-midwives provide constant companionship during labor, which I can't provide. I might have an operation going on."

Dr. Timothy Johnson, director of maternal/fetal medicine at Johns Hopkins University, says about nurse-midwives: "Nurse-midwives provide a safe alternative in routine obstetrical care. . . . There are good statistics to suggest that nurse-midwives are safe and cost effective. They know when to transfer care appropriately. The quality assurance and peer review of ACNM is high quality. . . . There's good scientific data to support the safety of nurse-midwives."

Some physicians, he said, do not understand that it is standard for certified nurse-midwives to practice in collaboration with doctors. Doctors who have never worked with nurse-midwives themselves may also not know that nurse-midwives have rigid standards for training and guidelines for collaborative practice with physicians. But as more young doctors work with nurse-midwives in obstetrical training programs they are learning the advantages of teamwork between the two groups of professionals.

"I'm an obstetrician and I like to deliver babies," Dr. Johnson said. "I'm happy to take care of low-risk women. But nurse-midwives have more time to educate their patients, to talk to them, to be with them during labor. They provide more personal care."

Doctors who work with nurse-midwives say other physicians should acknowledge that women and families are entitled to make choices about their own care; and that doctors should be open-minded, within safe standards, to providing the care that meets families' needs.

"Nurse-midwives have skills and training, they have

THE WORKING ARRANGEMENTS

Nurse-midwives can be found in a variety of working arrangements:

• *Private practices, owned by nurse-midwives.* Nurse-midwives provide all prenatal care and assistance in labor and birth, and contract with a physician who provides care if a woman develops complications. Births usually take place in a nearby hospital. In some practices, the nurse-midwives also attend home births, or do home births only, with a consulting physician available.

• *Private practices owned by physicians who employ nurse-midwives.* This increasingly popular model for practice allows women flexibility in choosing a doctor or nurse-midwife. A woman whose pregnancy is healthy and normal could receive all of her care from a nurse-midwife. Women generally give birth in a hospital.

• *Birth centers owned by nurse-midwives, physicians, or a hospital.* Women receive prenatal care and give birth at the center, which may be free-standing or part of a hospital. Nurse-midwives are the main caregivers at most birth centers, with consultation and referral available from physicians who have admitting privileges at a nearby hospital.

• *University hospitals.* Nurse-midwives may be employees of the obstetrical department or faculty members who may help educate physicians in training. Their consulting physicians may also be faculty members.

• *Health Maintenance Organizations.* Nurse-midwives on staff may be the primary caregivers throughout the pregnancy and hospital delivery for a healthy mother, with consultation provided by the HMO's physicians.

• *Public health departments and hospitals.* Nurse-midwives see women in prenatal clinics and are employed by hospitals to attend births.

good judgment and they know their bounds," said Dr. Julian Saffron, of Washington, D.C., who works with nurse-midwives in his private practice and provides consulting services to another practice run by nurse-midwives. "They have the knowledge and the skills to do it, and they do it well."

"Of course it's competition, but that's healthy," he said of the growing popularity of nurse-midwives. "There's enough room for me and for them and for other people too."

THE PROUD HISTORY OF A
MODERN PROFESSION

Although midwives of varied training have been delivering babies in the United States since the earliest settlers arrived, professional nurse-midwifery did not begin until the 1920s. Soon after the turn of the century, concern arose in the U.S. about high rates of maternal and infant death. Two groups, The Children's Bureau in Washington, D.C., and The Maternity Center Association in New York, perceived a link between infant death and lack of prenatal care. They began sending public health nurses into the community to instruct pregnant women in caring for themselves and their babies.

At about the same time, a nurse from Kentucky, Mary Breckenridge, traveled to England and France, where she observed the role that professionally trained midwives played in maternity care. She attended a British school of nurse-midwifery and in 1925 brought some of her British colleagues back with her to eastern Kentucky. There they rode horseback to visit pregnant women as part of the Frontier Nursing Service (FNS), which Breckenridge had

founded earlier in the twenties to bring health care to
people in isolated areas of the Appalachian mountains.

Meanwhile, maternal health experts began noting that
countries with excellent records in maternal and child health
used nurse-midwives. But there were no training programs in the U.S. At the urging of the Children's Bureau, the Maternity Center and the Lobenstine Clinic in
New York set up the country's first nurse-midwifery
school, which graduated its first class in 1933. A few years
later, the Frontier Nursing Service in Kentucky opened
its own nurse-midwifery school to fill the gap left when
the British nurse-midwives returned to serve their own
country during wartime. It continues as the oldest operating program in the U.S.

As more people recognized the role nurse midwives
could play in bringing high-quality, cost-effective care to
poor urban and rural women, more training programs
opened. The profession was on its way. In 1955, the
American College of Nurse-Midwifery was incorporated
in New Mexico to set national standards for education
and practice of nurse-midwives. In 1968 it merged with
the Kentucky-based American Association of Nurse-
Midwives, renaming itself the American College of Nurse-
Midwives, today's professional organization for nurse-
midwives.

During the decades just before nurse-midwifery began
in the United States, nearly all women—rich, poor or
middle class—gave birth at home. As had been the case
since colonial times, many births were attended by lay
midwives, women who usually had no formal training
but who were valued for their practical knowledge and
experience at the labor bed. Eventually, doctors got more
involved in maternity care and by the early 1900s, obstetrics evolved into a medical specialty. Birth moved from
the home to the hospital.

For women this was initially perceived as a huge step

forward, particularly with the advent of "twilight sleep," a combination of morphine and the amnesiac scopolamine, which made women feel little and remember little of the birth experience. Local or general anesthesia was given when the baby was close to delivery. Hospital birth seemed cleaner, safer, and less painful than birth at home and a woman had nurses, uninterrupted rest and relief from household duties. During the early years of hospitalization for childbirth, about 1915 to 1930, mortality rates rose, possibly due to inappropriate sterilization in hospitals and excessive intervention.[1] From 1936 to 1955, however, mortality rates dropped significantly as a standard of care was developed and new antibiotics helped fight infections and made cesarean sections much safer.[2]

The move to the hospital also medicalized birth, encouraging people to view it not as a normal occurrence, but rather as an illness, fraught with disasters waiting to happen. Interventions that were developed to save ailing mothers and babies were used routinely. Forceps, mind- and body-numbing drugs, and, later, an increasing rate of cesarean section improved some outcomes but added new risks for other mothers and babies. For instance, drugs that quieted laboring women and diminished the pain of childbirth also cast women into a fog, or knocked them out completely, making it difficult to push the baby out, thereby increasing the need for more drugs, forceps, and cesarean sections. Some women did not know they had given birth until waking hours later. Practices instituted for hospital efficiency altered the naturally slow pace of labor and birth, and many women did not experience the full joy that comes with birthing a new life.

Ironically, the lowered rate of maternal and infant death and the apparent safety of birth eventually prompted some mothers to question whether birth needed to be treated as a medical condition. By the early 1960s, a natural childbirth movement in the U.S. dovetailed with the nascent women's health movement. Within a decade, women were calling for more control over their medical care and their bodies. New books, pamphlets, and consciousness-raising sessions provided women with information that enabled them to become involved in health care decisions. They questioned practices that seemed more for the convenience of doctors and hospital staff than for the good of women and their babies.

Women wanted to be "awake and aware" for labor, not in a "twilight sleep" at the very hour a new baby would draw its first breath. They wanted to walk and squat during labor so gravity could help their baby, rather than lie on their backs with feet in stirrups. They wanted to breastfeed their newborns. And they wanted their families with them, not separated behind layers of glass. They wanted to redefine birth as an empowering experience that belonged to them, not one in which they gave up control to a medical system.

As women learned more, they began to see that pregnancy and childbirth could proceed in a normal, healthy fashion without medical interference. At the same time, routine childbirth was becoming more high-tech, as more technology was developed to gauge fetal health and detect abnormalities early. How could women draw upon the best of two worlds, the natural and the technological? Women sought allies in providing natural, family-centered births, without compromising safety.

They found nurse-midwives.

Suddenly, nurse-midwives were no longer caring only for poor women and children. They were in demand by middle class and more affluent women who wanted personalized, natural care. More hospitals began granting admitting privileges to nurse-midwives. Birth centers sprang up; more educational programs were established. In 1963, 275 nurse-midwives were working in the U.S., almost exclusively among low-income women. By 1976, their numbers leaped to 1,723 and by 1982 to 2,550—serving women across the economic spectrum. The demand has continued to grow as satisfied families spread the word.

During the 13-year period from 1975 to 1988, hospital births attended by nurse-midwives increased fivefold. In 1989, nurse-midwives attended 132,286 births in the U.S., representing 3.4 percent of all births that year. Of these, 125,451 were hospital births, 5,678 were in birth centers and 3,412 babies were born into the hands of nurse-midwives at home.[3]

Nurse-midwives in the U.S. are proud of their roots in public health, and glad to see their approach to safe and satisfying birth is now available to families across the economic spectrum. Certified nurse-midwives have technical training that sets them apart from their self-trained predecessors. Yet they cherish a spiritual connection to midwifery as it has been practiced throughout history. They are part of the tradition of women helping women, with special sensitivity, a sound theory base, and good common sense.

MIDWIFE MEANS "WITH WOMAN"— WHERE TO START

As early as Biblical times and in most cultures since, women have coached other women through labor. A certified nurse-midwife draws on that legacy of women-centered care, and adds to it her professional training.

More than anything, what nurse-midwives offer women is time. Whether it is time to answer all the questions in a prenatal visit or time to coax a slow labor, nurse-midwives are available. They have the time to sit with you and expertly guide you through the physical and emotional terrain of having a baby. Doctors acknowledge they have neither the time nor the personal inclination for long prenatal visits or to sit with a woman for ten or twelve hours of labor, rubbing her back and bolstering her confidence. Yet this personal support provides crucial enhancement to a woman's health and helps stave off medical complications.

The role of nurse-midwives continues to evolve. The distribution of nurse-midwives across the U.S. is uneven, with the highest concentration in places where consumer demand has been greatest, or doctors most accommodating. California has as many as four hundred Certified Nurse-Midwives (CNMs); Idaho has only six, spread across five cities. Nurse-midwife options vary greatly from one community to the next, and even within a single city, depending on the personality and preferences of the nurse-midwives and the willingness of doctors to work with them. Few communities offer the wide array of midwife arrangements possible, but if parents look, they will be able to find safe, personal and family-centered care with a nurse-midwife in most cities and towns.

This book describes nurse-midwives at work, showing how their approach is applied throughout pregnancy and childbirth. It will help you decide whether nurse-midwife care is right for you, and whether you are right for a nurse-midwife. The stories of nurse-midwives, mothers, and their families will describe what it is like to have a baby with a nurse-midwife. Separate chapters on various birth settings—hospital, birthing center and home—describe each experience, and suggest tips and questions to ask as you shop for care. Other chapters will answer your questions about the practical side of nurse-midwife care: safety statistics, costs and insurance coverage.

Safe, personal and family-centered care is your right as a parent. Whatever the birth setting or type of practice, nurse-midwives share a love of their calling and a zest for helping women through the work and wonder of child-birth. They are there to minimize concern and to maxi-mize good health and joy. Nurse-midwives take genuine pride in helping you find the strength and confidence to develop and birth a magnificent baby.

2.

NINE MONTHS:

Prenatal Care with a
Nurse-Midwife

*"The minute I started with the midwives, I knew
this was just great. It just felt very comfortable
. . . I felt like I was sitting talking to a friend."*
—KAREN, A MOTHER

IT WASN'T THAT Karen was so set on having her second
baby with a midwife. But after she moved from Manhattan to Brooklyn, she did not like the long subway ride
back to the doctor she used when her first child was born.
Neighbors told her about the nurse-midwives who worked
with an obstetrician just a few blocks from her new
apartment. The hospital where women delivered was close,
too.

During her first visit with a nurse-midwife, Karen was
convinced. The office was arranged so that the whole visit
could take place in one room. Her daughter could play
by the sofa where Karen and the nurse-midwife talked
before they moved over to the examining table. "There
was no waiting for the doctor to come, it was just very

relaxed," Karen said. "Right away, I just felt very different than I did at a doctor's office."

Women go to nurse-midwives for a variety of reasons.
Some are first-time mothers with clear ideas of what they
want in childbirth. Some feel their care in prior childbirth
experiences lacked warmth and support. Others heard
about a friend's good experience with a nurse-midwife.
Still others begin care with a nurse-midwife simply because it is convenient or is what their HMO or clinic offers.

Regardless of why women go to nurse-midwives, what
they find most satisfying is the rapport that develops with
the practitioner. As Karen learned, that rapport extends
beyond just one nurse-midwife. Although she rotated
among several nurse-midwives in the same practice for
prenatal visits, it was so clear they shared the same approach that Karen instantly felt comfortable with each one.

During the prenatal months, a nurse-midwife's goal is
to keep you and your growing baby healthy, and to help
you prepare physically and emotionally for labor. She does
that by education, by advising you on caring for yourself
and by instilling realistic expectations of pregnancy and
birth. She takes time to listen to you and pays attention
to the concerns that are particular to you and your pregnancy. She trusts you to know your body and your needs
and has the sharp clinical eye and experience with women
necessary to identify problems. Most of all, she commu-
nicates with you. She works *with* you to keep you at your
best.

THE FIRST VISIT

Even before the first prenatal appointment, some nurse-
midwives answer questions about their approach and
practice arrangement by phone. Most midwives ask ques-

tions that might reveal right away whether you have a medical condition that would rule you out for care in their practice. Many large nurse-midwife practices hold orientations so parents can become acquainted with their philosophy and see the place of birth before they sign up for care. Birth centers frequently have these group orientations; other practices hold orientations in the hospitals where their mothers deliver so you can tour the maternity and newborn facilities while you learn the particulars of the midwifery practice. These sessions hold no obligation, and are offered with the assumption that many parents want to comparison shop for the care that suits them best.

Ideal maternity care begins before conception, when the nurse-midwife advises you to create a good environment for conception by avoiding smoking, drinking, and drugs and staying close to your ideal weight. She also does initial health screenings. The first visit to a nurse-midwife, either preconception or after pregnancy has been confirmed, lasts longer than subsequent visits, and may range from one to two hours. It includes a standard set of questions and exams that would be part of your first prenatal visit, regardless of whether you were seeing a doctor or nurse-midwife. The nurse-midwife seeks as complete a medical history as you are able to give: your gynecological and obstetrical history; past illnesses and hospitalizations; medications; health habits and family history. Many midwives pay particular attention to your mother's obstetrical history, as it may offer clues to what lies ahead for you. The midwife is taught to test for immunity to German measles, which can lead to birth defects if contracted during pregnancy. Other genetic tests may be included.

Other checks done at this first visit normally include blood pressure; a Pap smear for cancer; a blood screening for blood type and to make sure your blood is not anemic; tests for gonorrhea and syphilis. The midwife usually examines your heart, lungs, abdomen, and breasts; records your height and weight; and checks for varicose veins and swelling. These indicators help her to assess your general health and serve as a base for comparison throughout the pregnancy. She also normally asks the date of your last menstruation to estimate your expected delivery date—roughly thirty-eight weeks after conception, or forty weeks after your last menstrual period. She also assesses the size and shape of your pelvis and performs an internal exam to check your cervix and uterus for signs of pregnancy and to check the health of pelvic organs. She also measures the uterus to confirm the date of the pregnancy.

Nurse-midwives normally accept for care only women without any medical conditions that could affect the likelihood of having a normal, healthy pregnancy. The definition of normal varies from one practice to the next, often depending on the arrangement between the nurse-midwife and consulting physician. In an HMO, clinic, or university hospital practice, for instance, criteria may be more flexible because a doctor is usually just down the hall if a consultation is needed.

The health evaluation of a first pregnancy visit with a nurse-midwife is much the same as it would be with a doctor. The differences come in how much time a nurse-midwife spends talking with you, and in her attitude toward you and your pregnancy. As Karen was pleased to find, midwives set up their offices with your physical and emotional comfort in mind. You first will meet the nurse-midwife with your clothes on, in a comfortable office, with a minimum of waiting time. After her checklist of questions and exams has been exhausted, she does not end the visit there. She talks with you, answering questions about midwifery, her practice, and what you can expect from her during pregnancy and labor. She begins finding out what the pregnancy means to you, how your family is responding, and how you are coping. Getting to know you as a person—you and your pregnancy together—is one of her first steps in becoming your partner for the mutual goal of a comfortable pregnancy and a healthy birth.

Even at that first visit, interspersed with the exams and discussion, a nurse-midwife is likely to begin teaching you about your pregnancy: to explain what each test or exam is for; to educate you about what is going on inside your body; to make clear that you can define your own pregnancy and can take responsibility for the new life forming inside you. Nutritional needs, exercise suggestions, books or articles to read are all likely topics during a first visit and are part of the expertise and guidance that a nurse-midwife offers.

WHO YOU WILL SEE AT EACH VISIT

During pregnancy, nurse-midwives tend to follow the same prenatal schedule as most doctors as long as all signs are normal: office visits once a month for the first 28 weeks; every 2 or 3 weeks from 28 weeks to 36 weeks; and then every 1 to 2 weeks until the baby is born. However, some women may be seen on a more flexible schedule, determined by the health needs of the mother and fetus. If you are healthy you will have fewer visits than a woman who is not.

Whom you see at each visit depends on the structure of the practice in which your midwife (or midwives) works. These are some common arrangements of midwifery practices, and how they work for prenatal care and the birth day:

Solo practices: A nurse-midwife in solo practice will see you herself for all prenatal visits. An advantage of this arrangement is that repeated contact with the same nurse-midwife enhances the bond that develops by the time you go into labor. And you know she will be the one to help you deliver your baby. But as with any solo practitioner, if she is ill or on vacation when you are ready to deliver, you may end up with someone you have never met.

Group practices: In many nurse-midwife partnerships or group practices, women see the same nurse-midwife for the majority of prenatal visits and refer to her as "my midwife." In other practices, women rotate through the group. In either case, it is likely you will be scheduled for at least one visit with each nurse-midwife so that you will be acquainted with whomever is on call when your labor begins. An advantage is that you have a larger support system, and perhaps the possibility of choosing care with the nurse-midwife you like best.

Doctor-owned: An increasingly popular arrangement is for doctors to employ nurse-midwives to work in their practices. Some women choose to see only a nurse-midwife (or rotate among midwives in the practice) for the entire pregnancy and delivery. Other women choose to see only a doctor. A woman may also alternate visits between a doctor and midwife, and decide by the last trimester whom she prefers for labor and delivery. This type of practice is advantageous for a woman who wants nurse-midwife care, yet knows that if a complication develops she will remain in the same practice. Other women avoid this arrangement, feeling that a nurse-midwife within a doctor's office may not have complete freedom to follow her own philosophy.

HMOs and clinics: In large Health Maintenance Organizations and clinics, you may see a different nurse-midwife for each prenatal visit. Most groups, however, try to keep you with the same midwife for most of your visits. The midwife on duty will attend your labor and delivery. Although rotating among nurse-midwives is not the ideal situation for creating a bond, women are comfortable knowing that all practitioners in the group share the same approach.

Whether you see a doctor at all prenatally will depend partly on the agreement between your midwife and her consulting physician. Some arrangements require each woman to see the doctor at least once or twice during pregnancy. Under other agreements, women who have no complications do not see the doctor at all unless they want to. Many mothers who are healthy throughout pregnancy find no need to meet the doctor. But a small percentage of them—some 5 to 10 percent—develop complications during labor that require a doctor's attention.

PRENATAL VISITS

On visits after your first one, a nurse-midwife is likely to take your blood pressure and may check your urine for protein and sugar, just as a physician would do. She also typically records your weight and measures your belly to gauge fetal growth and listens to the fetal heartbeat. With her hands, a nurse-midwife also becomes acquainted with you and your baby. By feeling from the outside, she gauges the size and shape of your uterus; by the seventh month, she can tell the size and position of the fetus.

It usually is not thought necessary to perform an internal exam after the first visit, so many midwives avoid the examining table for a more relaxing environment. At one California home birth practice, for instance, each nurse-midwife's office looks more like a sitting room than an examination room, with a large, soft couch covered in floral print, a desk and homelike sink. After a woman has weighed herself and given a urine sample, she lies on the couch and pushes her clothes aside so the nurse-midwife can measure her belly. Then she sits back up for the remainder of the visit, often with the nurse-midwife sitting alongside her. An examining table is in a small room next door if an internal exam is needed.

Nurse-midwives allow young children, spouses and prospective grandparents to come along. In some practices, it is not uncommon for some spouses to attend nearly every prenatal visit. In other practices, partners are encouraged to come to particular visits. If young siblings come along, nurse-midwives involve them in the exam, asking the youngsters to "help" measure their mother's belly, take blood pressure or listen to the fetal heartbeat.

In concert with the philosophy that a woman should be active in her own care, the expectant mother may begin the rudiments of each visit on her own. At the Maternity Center Association in New York, the oldest free-standing birth center in the U.S., a woman begins each prenatal visit by retrieving her own chart, recording her weight, and testing her own urine sample for protein and sugar using dipsticks and a color-coded chart. Meanwhile, she has time to think about the note that the nurse-midwife has attached to her chart, explaining something that will be discussed later in the visit. Expectant mothers find they like participating that way. Being included in their own care, with regular review of their own charts, makes women feel more confident in themselves and in their nurse-midwives. There are no secrets; mother and nurse-midwife embark on the pregnancy together.

A typical prenatal visit with a nurse-midwife lasts a half hour, two or three times as long as some physicians allot. That extra time is spent educating you about what is happening inside your body and how to keep you and your growing baby healthy. The more you understand, the better you will be able to care for yourself.

A nurse-midwife fosters the attitude that pregnancy should be nurtured. She encourages you to love your pregnancy the way you will love your baby. It may indeed be difficult to love a pregnancy during those times when it gives you morning sickness and exhaustion in return. But tips for coping with these inconveniences, and perpetual encouragement of good health habits, help keep mother and baby on a positive track.

NUTRITION AND WEIGHT GAIN

A cornerstone of good health during pregnancy is nutrition. Some women have a very clear idea of what it means to eat the recommended 80 grams of protein daily; others are mystified. A nurse-midwife explains nutritional needs during pregnancy, working with your tastes, preferences, and allergies to make sure you are getting adequate calories and nutrients for your baby to grow. She also advises you on vitamins.

Nurse-midwives tend not to have strict rules on weight gain. The Institutes of Medicine's recommendation is for pregnant women to gain 30 to 33 pounds—or slightly more if underweight to begin with. A midwife is also likely to take into account your body type and weight gain with previous pregnancies. She encourages you to listen to your body and do what feels comfortable as long as you are

getting adequate nutrition. If you are particularly concerned about not carrying much extra weight after pregnancy, your nurse-midwife can guide you to adequate
nutrition without an overload of calories. The approach
is always personalized; each body accommodates pregnancy differently.

One first-time mother, for instance, who never could
tip a scale beyond 99 pounds no matter how she tried,
was proud of the extra effort she made to eat nutritious
foods as soon as she became pregnant. But her doctor
scolded her for gaining 11 pounds during her first trimester, saying she was gaining ahead of schedule and would
have trouble taking it off later.

"I was so offended," she said. "I thought I should be
congratulated!"

The midwives she saw later during that pregnancy did
not question her weight gain, 35 pounds, which was appropriate for a normal pregnancy. Sure enough, after the
birth, her old body chemistry returned. She dropped back
to below 100 pounds. With her second baby, the very
same thing happened: a 35-pound weight gain, quickly
shed.

Listen to your body, a nurse-midwife tells you. And
your nurse-midwife will listen to you.

EXERCISE

If aerobics class helped keep you fit and sane before pregnancy, you probably will not be asked to give it up, although your midwife may suggest modifications. She will
encourage you not to drive yourself as hard as in prepreg-
nancy days. Your body will give you clues.

Fitness-conscious Jane, the New York lawyer who
shopped so extensively for maternity care, chose her nurse-

midwives in part because they would not discourage her from continuing aerobics. To her surprise, however, Jane found herself so exhausted during early pregnancy she lost interest in the gym. As her early weight gain edged toward the upper limits of the normal range, however, her nurse-midwife was concerned that the halt to Jane's exercise regimen had slowed down her metabolism. She suggested Jane push herself a little and get to the gym. Remember, a midwife's goal is to help you retain your normal state of health throughout the pregnancy. Sure enough, after Jane dragged herself to a few classes, her energy level picked up, and her weight gain slowed to a more suitable rate for her stage of pregnancy.

PRENATAL TESTING

Rapidly changing technology and personal values make prenatal testing among the most difficult issues parents face during pregnancy. Testing includes ultrasound pictures and genetic and blood screenings that can indicate fetal abnormalities. With some obstetricians, these tests are routine. However, testing involves pros and cons; many tests present a risk to fetus or mother. Nurse-midwives regard prenatal testing as they do any technological intervention: valuable when it provides useful information that could not be learned otherwise and when the potential benefits outweigh the risks.

A nurse-midwife may recommend a test if there are signs or family history of an abnormality. Otherwise, the decision of whether to test is left up to parents. In either case, a nurse-midwife explains the benefits and risks of each test. For some parents, the decision to test may be the first taste of the responsibility of having a child. The nurse-midwife answers questions and helps parents make their decision. She also explains, in advance, what parents' options would be given possible test results. Any discussion of genetic testing includes your attitudes on terminating a pregnancy. Nurse-midwives do not perform abortions, but they may be involved in counseling and care before and after the procedure. (See Chapter 4 for more details on testing.)

Nurse-midwife Barbara Brennan of New York considers prenatal testing within the scope of the guidance she offers pregnant women. If she is uncertain about when a baby is due, for instance, she may recommend a sonogram so she will know months later whether labor is beginning prematurely. But if there is no medical reason to seek out more information, most testing decisions are left to parents.

"Sonogram, chorionic villus sampling, amnio, genetic counseling—it is the parents' decision to make," she said. "But we make it available to them so they can make that decision."

NO QUESTION TOO SILLY OR TOO SMALL

"You fill a mother's cup up to the top," goes an old midwife saying. "And then she has something more to pour out to her babe."

The adage applies well to modern nurse-midwives. Pregnant women find themselves thirsting for information, and questions pop up daily that seem almost too silly to ask. But midwives are there to answer those questions, as normal, they believe, as pregnancy itself.

"With physicians you sometimes get the feeling you've asked a dumb question," said Sarah, the South Florida mother who had three children with nurse-midwife Marilynn Wender. "But with Marilynn I never felt that I asked a dumb question. She had the attitude that the more I knew, the better it would be for my pregnancy, the better for me and for my baby. I felt she was genuinely interested in me."

Three mothers from New York, who gave birth with three different nurse-midwifery practices, felt the same openness:

• Laura, an executive secretary, chose nurse-midwives because she liked their philosophy toward childbirth and was pleased at some of the side benefits. "With a first pregnancy you have a lot of questions—you know, 'Should I be eating Ring Dings?' " Her friends had complained about five-minute office visits with their obstetricians that left many questions unanswered. Laura never had that problem. "If I ever had a question they always called me back, and the office visits were always a half-hour long," she said. "They'd ask me if I had questions. They spent a lot of time with me. I really liked that."

• Jane and Danny are accomplished professionals, accustomed to dealing with complex matters. But in the business of having a baby they knew they were novices, and they appreciated the way their midwives answered their questions without belittling their concerns and fears.

"These nurse-midwives may have delivered twelve million babies, but this is my first one and it's a unique experience to me. Why should any question or feeling I have be treated with anything less than the respect or full answer it deserves, simply because the caregiver has answered it four hundred times?" Jane said. "The nurse-midwives made very clear that they realized this was the first time I was going through this, I had no idea what childbirth would be like, and I would not be treated in a hurry."

"You wouldn't elicit a frown or a face that said, 'that's a dumb question' or 'don't ask that kind of stuff,' " Danny added. He liked the feeling of full disclosure from the midwives, and he never felt that the clock was running.

"We had appointments that lasted fifteen minutes. Other times we were there for a full hour if we had questions or wanted to talk about something. We never had a sense of anybody looking at a watch and saying, 'Hey, I got a roomful of people, can you move it along?' None of that."

• Patience and respect are important no matter how many children a mother has had. Each pregnancy is unique. By her second pregnancy, Karen, the Brooklyn mother who changed from an obstetrician to nurse-midwives for convenience' sake, felt like an old hand at childbirth. She figured pregnancy meant "basically, take your vitamins and eat." Although she liked her obstetrician and felt comfortable with him, the nurse-midwives were a nice change.

"I felt more of a time pressure with him, he was more businesslike," she said. "I felt like I had to come up with questions fast, get the answer, boom-boom-boom, get in and out. He answered my questions and I liked what he said, it's just that I felt like I had to be efficient and not waste his time. He was a busy guy."

With her doctor, Karen chose her words carefully, always feeling that she had to be "a good patient." The nurse-midwives brought out a different side of her. "I could be relaxed, I could be funny, I could be me," she said. "I didn't have to be the good patient. They would accept me no matter what I said, no matter what I did. They were there for me."

THE HOLISTIC APPROACH

During the prenatal months, your nurse-midwife looks at pregnancy's full range of physical implications, then beyond, to its links with your emotional state. Holistic is the word frequently used to describe this approach.

Denise is a hospital social worker from suburban Detroit who had her first daughter with a doctor and the second with a nurse-midwife. The doctor's care, she said, focused "entirely on the waist down." But there were other aspects of childbirth that needed attention. For instance, she told the doctor that she planned to breastfeed, but he gave little instruction. As it turned out, Denise initially had difficulty, as some women do. A little assistance and early preparation might have saved her much frustration.

The next birth was with a nurse-midwife who focused on pregnancy in its fullest sense—mind, body and emotions. Beyond providing helpful answers to Denise's questions, she anticipated other concerns.

"She initiated conversations about sex, about maintaining the marital relationship during pregnancy, asking about your emotional state," Denise said. "Even when I didn't have questions prepared, she would say, 'At this point in your pregnancy, these are some of the things you may be experiencing.' She was talking about physically, emotionally, marital relationship-wise—the entire thing. She wanted you to be totally aware and involved in the pregnancy. There was time set aside and if you didn't take advantage of it, she would. For you. It wasn't just a checkup."

A nurse-midwife knows how emotional strain can have a physical impact on pregnancy. Elsie Wilson, a nurse-midwife who has worked in Kentucky, Africa, and Florida, suspects that when a woman answers "yes" to every query about the myriad of physical discomforts that may accompany pregnancy, it may be a sign that something else is troubling her.

"I sit down with her, look her straight in the eye, even reach out and touch her, and say 'Now what's really going on? What's frightening you, what's bothering you?' " Wilson said. "And she'll probably break down in tears and tell you she had a fight with her partner, or she's worried that something she did in the past is going to reflect on this pregnancy. And you have an opportunity to help her through that situation. Sometimes, you just have to take time to get beyond the surface."

When it comes to the complex emotions and mood swings of pregnancy, a nurse-midwife is an expert. She can help you address psychological factors that may be contributing to your nausea or rising blood pressure. But she will not try to play therapist. If she detects a serious emotional problem she will make an appropriate referral. What she offers is a little help navigating the turbulence that imminent motherhood can bring.

TOUGH LOVE FOR SARAH

Sarah, from South Florida, learned how far a nurse-midwife's concern could take her when she became pregnant with her third child. When she was pregnant with her first child ten years earlier, Sarah had made an appointment with an obstetrician, only to find that nurse-midwife Marilynn Wender tended all uncomplicated pregnancies in his practice. Sarah loved the experience. Marilynn's encouragement to give he baby a good start even led her to cut out cigarettes by her fourth month, a difficult feat for someone who had smoked two packs a day for ten years.

During Sarah's second pregnancy, she cut back on her daily cigarettes, but could not give them up completely. It happened to be a stressful time in Sarah's personal life, and Marilynn helped her through it, as well as through a difficult labor.

By Sarah's third pregnancy at age thirty-five, she could not imagine giving birth without Marilynn. But the nurse-midwife she counted on so much shocked her with an ultimatum: she would not accept Sarah for maternity care again unless she quit smoking. Marilynn was concerned that smoking contributed to the low birthweights of Sarah's first two children, and she felt that a woman who had smoked heavily for twenty years was too risky for her. Sarah promised to cut out cigarettes. But Marilynn knew Sarah could be wily; to keep her honest, she vowed to check her blood for nicotine at each prenatal visit. Sarah was shaken by Marilynn's harsh approach, but it worked. She resorted to acupuncture, kicked her habit and never resumed smoking.

"I probably would have been offended if a doctor said that to me, threatened me that way," said Sarah, who had been trying to quit for ten years. She knew the adverse affects of smoking on a fetus, but felt truly addicted.

Stern treatment from someone whose opinion she valued was the motivation Sarah needed. And Marilynn knew Sarah well enough to be confident in taking a hard-line approach.

"Marilynn's threat not to deliver my baby was the only thing that could have gotten me to quit smoking," Sarah said. "I wanted Marilynn to bring my baby into the world."

That baby, Sarah is proud to say, weighed 8 pounds, 11 3/4 ounces at birth, a healthy two pounds more than her first two children.

PREPARATION FOR LABOR—EMOTIONAL

Being prepared for labor, both physically and emotionally, is your best coping tool. In prenatal visits, a nurse-midwife explains step-by-step what will happen once labor begins: how your body and your baby's will adapt to the strains of labor, and what you may feel at each point. She talks about what will be going on around you, be it in a hospital, birthing center, or home. Media images, "war stories" from friends and family, prior experiences and a woman's own fears may add up to considerable, and understandable, trepidation about labor. A midwife's goal is to help a woman feel confident that pregnancy and labor are designed by nature to work.

"You have to begin in the prenatal visits to get women to talk about what they are afraid of," said LaRita Evans, a nurse-midwife who has worked in Utah for fifteen years. "If you really believe that pregnancy is a normal function of a woman's body, you convey that. It makes a huge difference in the whole outcome of the pregnancy."

If a woman has a particular concern, simple as a fear of needles or complex as not being ready for motherhood, those sometimes hidden fears can impede labor. A pregnant woman's concerns, rational or not, are real to her. A nurse-midwife tries to diminish those anxieties through relaxed discussions early in pregnancy so that when labor begins, the woman is free to follow nature's flow. Working with nature's process in labor, not fighting it, helps labor proceed as smoothly as possible.

Nurse-midwife Nancy McNeese, who owns a birthing center outside Los Angeles, notes that fear and anxiety can block natural pain-inhibiting chemicals that ease labor. One of her goals is to understand, and resolve, the "emotional baggage" a woman may bring to labor long before the first contraction.

"When we're excited or afraid our body reacts," she said. "Childbirth is a natural, normal process. But if someone has a lot of things that are blocking that natural, normal process, the woman is going to get tense. And when you have a fear-tension-pain-cycle in labor, it is hard to break and the woman gets very, very tired."

PREPARATION FOR LABOR—PHYSICAL

The female body is built to produce a baby, and you can help by giving nature every advantage. If your muscles, lungs, and heart are accustomed to exertion, you will have more endurance during labor, which could make a cesarean less likely. Good muscle tone makes it easier to squat during labor, an efficient way to move things along. During pregnancy, nurse-midwives recommend moderate exercise such as walking or slow swimming to keep up muscle tone and endurance, even for women who did not exercise much before.

Your midwife will be able to show you how to do Kegel exercises—and nag you plenty about doing them!—to strengthen the pelvic floor muscles that are important in labor. You will thank her later, especially after delivery when resuming the Kegels may help to restore muscle tone to the perineum and rectum.

Some nurse-midwives show women how to soften and stretch their own perineal tissue during the weeks before birth. Massaging the area with oils or gels, they believe, increases flexibility and ability to stretch, avoiding a cut or tear. A 1986 study found that women who massaged the perineum at least four times weekly during the final six weeks of pregnancy had a lower rate of episiotomies and tears than those who did not.[1] Not all nurse-midwives agree that perineal massage is effective, but at the very least it accustoms you to the pressure and stinging you may feel as your baby's head is born.

In addition to the informal instruction nurse-midwives offer during prenatal care, they expect first-time parents to take childbirth classes and suggest refresher classes for veterans. Nurse-midwives leave it up to parents to choose the method of childbirth classes they would like to attend i.e., Bradley, Lamaze, or whatever is offered at the local hospital or birth center. More important than learning a particular method, mothers and their partners should learn the relaxation and breathing techniques taught in all classes. Once labor begins, a nurse-midwife often cannot tell which type of class a couple took, but invariably, laboring women and their partners take something they learned in class and adapt it to their needs.

As labor draws closer, a nurse-midwife generally encourages rest. That way, no matter what time labor begins you will have a reserve of energy to help your body work more efficiently. Women who are unable to take time off from jobs or a heavy household burden are encouraged to seek help from friends or relatives. Those accustomed to long work days and full social schedules are urged to slow down.

Nurse-midwife Barbara Brennan in New York tells women to consider themselves in training for the most grueling athletic contest: "If you were going to run a marathon, you would say, 'Gee, I better eat well, rest, keep everyone off the phone, and not have a lot of visitors so I can go into it feeling good,' Labor may not happen at nine o'clock in the morning after a good night's sleep. It may happen at three a.m. It just makes sense to be rested."

Ali, a Los Angeles mother who had two babies at home used the same road-race analogy for childbirth. "If you're going to run a marathon, you train for it," she said. "Labor is more strenuous. My nurse-midwives stress taking care of yourself and preparing. It seems like the more you can do for yourself, the better." Like many women, Ali found it empowering to take charge of her pregnancy.

WHAT IF . . .?

As we've said before, normal birth is a nurse-midwife's expertise. When there are signs in a pregnancy of an irregularity, she consults with the physician in accordance with the standards of her profession. If the condition warrants, the woman is transferred to an obstetrician's care.

For some complications, such as pregnancy-induced high blood pressure and mild diabetes, a nurse-midwife may continue as the primary caregiver after consulting with the doctor. Doctors and midwives call such an arrangement "co-management." Any woman with a complication that requires birth by cesarean section is transferred to the doctor's care. Sometimes, though, the nurse-midwife continues the prenatal care with the understanding that the physician will perform the cesarean birth.

Your nurse-midwife explains in advance that if certain situations arise during pregnancy or labor, birth plans will have to be altered. You may not care to think about complications, but it is worth paying attention to these details so you will have realistic expectations if a complication develops.

"I tell them, but women think they are just not going to have a high-risk pregnancy, they just are not going to have a C-section. So they just don't hear it," said nurse-midwife Lisa Summers, who has worked in Texas, New York, and Maryland. "They want to hear all the good, exciting stuff. They want to hear about cosmic birth. They don't want to hear about operating rooms."

Sometimes a complication emerges after a woman has developed considerable confidence and trust in her nurse-midwife. She may want the midwife to continue to care for her, with the kind of birth they had planned. But as Denise found, that is not always possible.

Early in her first pregnancy, the hospital social worker from suburban Detroit developed a rapid increase in blood pressure. Her condition posed a serious enough risk to mother and fetus that her nurse-midwife said she should transfer to a physician. Denise wanted very much to have her baby with Thersa, the nurse-midwife she had chosen. But Denise learned that a nurse-midwife takes no chances:

"I was so disappointed that I was not going to be able to continue with Thersa, disappointed to the point of almost willing to risk not going to the doctor," Denise said. "Of course she would not have allowed that." Although Denise transferred to the doctor, she drew on the self-confidence that Thersa had begun to nurture. With her next pregnancy, Denise's blood pressure remained manageable enough that she stayed with her nurse-midwife for the pregnancy and labor.

BREECH BABIES—A LITTLE EXTRA HELP

Most babies position themselves head down by the eighth month, an accommodation by nature for the easiest delivery. But some babies remain upright, in less convenient "breech" positions. Whether they are buttocks-first with legs tucked or shooting upward, or upright with one foot dangling, breech babies can be difficult to deliver vaginally. For babies lying sideways, in transverse position, vaginal birth is nearly impossible.

Many obstetricians prepare for cesarean section if the baby is in the breech position toward the end of pregnancy. Nurse-midwives, however, wait until labor to see if the baby turns before calling in the doctor for a cesarean.

If your baby is in a breech position, a nurse-midwife generally works patiently with you toward the end of pregnancy to get the baby to turn so you can have a vaginal birth. She may encourage you to lie on your back with feet and hips elevated at an angle, on a sit-up board or slanted ironing board, for twenty minutes daily. This often nudges the baby to turn into the head-down vertex position.

Nancy, the Miami lawyer whose birth is described at the beginning of Chapter 1, was thirty weeks pregnant when she learned that her baby was breech. Her nurse-midwives would not deliver a breech baby, and Nancy very much wanted to avoid a cesarean. Twice daily, she lay with her hips elevated and massaged her belly. Two weeks into this routine, she was lying in bed with a pillow under her hips one evening, when the baby turned. Nancy actually felt it. It was a wonderful victory, and a cherished moment of feeling very much in touch with her baby.

"She may have turned around anyways, but I felt like *I* was doing something," Nancy said. "I was thrilled."

Another option for a breech is fetal version—turning the baby manually from outside the mother's belly before labor using ultrasound as a guide to avoid compressing the umbilical cord. This requires an experienced pair of hands, and only a few doctors and nurse-midwives are skilled at it.

EACH PREGNANCY HAS A LIFE OF ITS OWN

Every pregnancy is unique, and a nurse-midwife tailors her care accordingly. Some women need little nutritional guidance, but much emotional support. Others are confident about coping with a new baby, but panicked by the physical changes of pregnancy. A nurse-midwife makes an effort to learn and address each woman's specific needs.

Theresa, for instance, needed a lot of encouragement for her second pregnancy after the first ended in miscarriage. Remembering how insensitive her doctor seemed after the miscarriage, Theresa chose a nurse-midwife for her second pregnancy. She very much wanted that baby, and she was anxious and nervous. She was far away from the support of family and old friends, having moved from Florida to Minnesota before the first pregnancy. Her experienced nurse-midwife used just the right approach to reassure her.

"It was the encouragement, the way she treated my belly, the words she used," Theresa said. "I felt like I was being mothered, and that was just what I needed. She kept reminding me that things progress on their own."

Jane, on the other hand, needed a different approach. The New York lawyer felt confident through most of her pregnancy, barely curtailing her bustling work and social schedule. In her eighth month, a business trip to Houston came up, something that was important to her personally and professionally, but she knew most women avoid travel in the third trimester. She called one of her nurse-midwives and explained the situation. "I'm not going to go if you tell me there's any good reason not to go. But tell me, is there any medical reason?"

There was no distinct medical reason not to go, the nurse-midwife explained, except that if Jane got overtired, the exhaustion would be hard to shake late in pregnancy. And, in the unlikelihood that she went into labor early, she would be with strangers. Jane decided to go. Following her midwife's suggestion, she slowed her pace by staying an extra night. And, she took a copy of her medical chart and the phone numbers of a few Houston nurse-midwives just in case. She was glad her nurse-midwife was able to consider Jane's priorities when helping her make the decision.

"I wouldn't say she encouraged the trip but she didn't put a big damper on it," Jane said. "She had a strong sense that it was important to me. I went, I came back. I was very happy that I had done it. I felt very gratified professionally. I liked the fact that once again my nurse-midwife had been calm, not reactionary."

For first-time parents especially, it is difficult to know how you will respond to the huge changes brought on by pregnancy. But your midwife probably has seen a response like yours before, the same physical ailment or particular worry, and she helps you address it. Then, when those first few labor pains signal the beginning of the home stretch, you are physically healthy and emotionally prepared. And your midwife is there with you.

3.

STOPPING THE CLOCK:

Labor and Delivery

*"I had a wonderful labor, I loved it, I really did.
. . . It was like, this is what my body is supposed to be doing. It felt great. . . . The more
powerful the contraction, the more it hurt, the
more I thought: this is a powerful thing, my body
is doing what it's supposed to be doing, and I'm
that much closer to the baby."*
—ELIZABETH, A FIRST-TIME MOTHER

ELIZABETH'S DESCRIPTION OF labor is not one with which
every woman would agree. Not everyone copes as well
with the painful contractions of labor. But Elizabeth's attitude about the hours that culminated with the birth of
her son, Jonathan, mirrors a nurse-midwife's approach to
labor and birth: it is difficult work to bring a baby into
the world, but a woman's body is engineered just right
to handle the job.

During labor and birth a nurse-midwife follows the same
basic principles that guide prenatal care: birth is a natural,
healthy process that can occur on its own, but a skilled

nurse-midwife can make it easier, safer, and more comfortable. Details of the delivery vary depending on whether you are having your baby in a hospital, birth center, or at home, but the approach is the same.

In labor, you enter your own realm of time, no matter what the clock says. A nurse-midwife follows your cues and lets labor proceed at its own pace, yet is watchful for exceedingly slow progress that may signal a problem. During early labor, she helps you relax and gives you tips to cope, so you will be able to save your energy for the more difficult hours ahead. Once the contractions start coming fast and hard, she stays with you, offering what a woman in labor needs most: patience. She is beside you, monitoring you and your baby closely. Her keen attention, her training, and her experience in healthy birth mean that your nurse-midwife is likely to notice any problem at an early stage. She guides you through those miraculous hours that transform you from a pregnant woman to a mother with an infant nursing peacefully in your arms.

FIRST STAGE—EARLY LABOR

A nurse-midwife's calm and patience is apparent from that first phone call when you tell her you think labor is beginning. After a few questions to gauge that all is well, she says: "Wonderful! Go back to sleep. Turn on some relaxing music. Take a bath. Or a nap." If the contractions are just the Braxton-Hicks type that occur in the weeks preceding true labor, they stop once you are relaxed and still. But if contractions continue after the bath or nap, you know this is the real thing at last.

For nearly all women, and especially for first-time mothers, labor is a long process. Babies are rarely born within a few hours; births in elevators and taxicabs happen mostly on television. You usually have time to relax through the early hours of labor.

Nurse-midwives encourage women to remain at home as long as possible before coming to the hospital or birth center. Labor proceeds more quickly if a woman is comfortable, and most people are most comfortable in their own homes with their own couch, tub, and tea-kettle. No doubt, you will be excited and eager to get on with your final hours of pregnancy, but a midwife encourages you and your partner to get the rest you will need for later. You should eat something light and easy to digest to fuel your body. Liquids, especially fruit juice and herbal tea with honey, prevent dehydration and keep up your energy level. Those early contractions may seem strenuous, but they are scant compared to what lies ahead. You will have an advantage later if you are fortified and rested.

During those first few hours at home, your nurse-midwife keeps in close contact by phone. She asks if your bag of waters—the amniotic sac that surrounds the baby—has broken. (If so, she may suggest you shower rather than take a bath.) For some women, the gush or trickle of amniotic fluid when the waters break is the first sign that labor is beginning; for others the sac does not break until moments before the birth. Your midwife also asks about other signs of labor, such as increased mucus production and the frequency, strength, and duration of contractions. By listening carefully, she knows when you are entering the more active phase of labor.

JANE'S STORY

Jane, the New York City lawyer who shopped so rigorously before choosing a nurse-midwife, was close to the due date for her first child when a contraction jolted her awake at 3 a.m. She remembered what her nurse-midwives suggested when the first labor pains began: she poured a small glass of Bailey's Irish Cream, maneuvered herself into an easy chair, and relaxed. The contractions stopped.

Jane stayed home that day, Saturday, after calling her midwives and telling them about the start-and-stop pains. A few friends dropped by, and her husband lined up the three videos she had chosen to fill the hours of early labor. By Sunday, Jane was clearly in early labor, with erratic contractions. By the third movie, she could not follow the plot. Contractions commanded her attention.

Meanwhile, the midwife-on-call phoned her every few hours through the weekend. Jane was puzzled because her labor did not seem to follow the benchmarks in the books. She saw no signs of the mucus plug and her bag of waters did not break. Every labor is unique, her midwives assured. Hers was just going at its own pace.

By Monday, the contractions were still erratic, but much stronger. And the baby had turned around, leaving Jane with a horrendous backache. "Back labor," as it is called, usually means the baby is in the posterior position, with the back of its head tucked against the mother's lower backbone. Despite the discomfort, Jane felt at ease. She was with her husband, in her own home, and well cared for over the phone. Every six hours, one of the midwives called.

"Even before we went to the hospital I felt like the midwives were constantly with me," she said. "The whole time they were filled with incredibly good suggestions. When I had back labor, which was excruciatingly painful, they said to take a bath. It made a big difference. . . . If I had been with an obstetrician, I think I would have been in the hospital for three days."

Early Tuesday, Jane's contractions escalated in pain and

intensity. Jane knew it was time to go to the hospital. That afternoon, Allison was born.

EASIER TO REST AT HOME

Most women find it difficult to rest once they enter a hospital. Many find they are best off not arriving until labor takes so much concentration they hardly notice anything else. That is what Elizabeth, who had such a satisfying labor, found.

The day before the baby was born, however, was more unsettling. In her ninth month, Elizabeth was put on bed rest because of her high blood pressure. Then, around the time of her due date, her blood pressure rose so high that the midwife-doctor team admitted her to the hospital to keep close watch on her and the baby. A prostaglandin gel was applied to her cervix, to soften it and encourage labor, but the gel triggered strong prelabor contractions and vomiting. When Elizabeth's body finally calmed, noise on the ward and her unease at being there kept her from sleeping—by morning she was exhausted. She was given a choice: go home and return in twenty-four hours for a check on the baby, or induce labor in the hospital. Grateful for the choice, Elizabeth went home.

Back in her own apartment, Elizabeth relaxed and slept. Within hours, mild contractions began. Her husband Jim called their birth assistant to come to their apartment, as they had arranged. She made soup, and Elizabeth ate a small bowlful.

Comfortable in her own bedroom, Elizabeth felt able to manage the contractions better than she could in the hospital. She rested in between contractions, while the birth assistant listened to the baby's heartbeat on a fetal stethoscope.

"I didn't know if this was real labor or not," Elizabeth

recalled. "I was making all these noises, and the birth assistant would say 'Good!' And I'd make another noise and she'd say 'Good!' "

Finally, when the contractions came very close together, Elizabeth called her nurse-midwife and went back to the hospital—just in time to begin pushing.

Nurse-midwives do not have strict rules for how quickly labor must progress before they interfere to speed it up, as long as the baby's heartbeat and other key indicators are normal. Most do not set a time to artificially rupture membranes if the bag of waters has not broken on its own. And most do not set a guideline, as some hospitals do, that a woman must dilate at least one centimeter per hour or receive a labor-speeding drug such as Pitocin.

Audrey, a physician, gave birth to two sons with the same nurse-midwives as Elizabeth in Ann Arbor. She knew from her medical training that doctors and nurses are less likely than nurse-midwives to let labor proceed on its own.

"Doctors and nurses lose patience with a laboring woman," Audrey said. "They feel like, 'well, this patient is sitting in this bed, I ought to do something to them. I'm a doctor, I'm a nurse, I *do* things to patients. I don't just let them lie in bed or wander the hallways squatting and things like that.' "

If you are not in the care of a nurse-midwife, simply being in a hospital during early labor may increase the likelihood of medical intervention, such as labor-speeding drugs, when all you and your baby really need is a little time to allow nature to take its course.

KNOWING WHEN IT'S TIME

Because most early labors do not progress according to textbook descriptions, an experienced nurse-midwife helps determine where you are in labor. Nurse-midwives usually advise women to go to their hospital or birth center—or call the midwife if it is a home birth—when contractions occur about every three to five minutes and last a minute or so. That generally means the cervix has opened, or dilated, at least four centimeters and the most active stage of labor is underway. Many women do not have such regular contractions; others dilate more while contractions occur far apart; still others stall at a few centimeters for hours. When the cervix is dilated a full ten centimeters, the mother usually feels the urge to push the baby out.

For someone who has given birth before, labor proceeds more quickly. A second or third-time mom usually knows when she is ready to go to the hospital.

For first-time mothers, nurse-midwives have their own well-honed gauges to determine when a woman is entering active labor. Nurse-midwife Barbara Brennan asks a question as a contraction is reaching its height. If a first-time mother keeps chatting through the contraction, Barbara knows it is still early. Nurse-midwife Barbara Sellars listens for a certain "singing" through the breathing, which tells her that labor has escalated. Kay Johnson, a Houston nurse-midwife, calls it the "drop phone" sign: when contractions are powerful enough to make a first-time mother drop the phone, it is time for her to go to the hospital.

These rules-of-thumb, however, are personalized for each woman. Barbara Sellars learned through months of prenatal visits and a previous ectopic pregnancy that Roi was a stoic, not one to say much even during great discomfort. That is why when Roi's husband called a few hours into labor sounding panicked, Barbara suggested they meet at the hospital, even though Roi's breathing was still quiet. Barbara preferred to err on the side of caution. Sure enough, Roi was dilated only two centimeters. Barbara sent her back home.

"Within two hours, I was singing," Roi remembered

with a laugh months afterwards. "We went to the hospital and by then I was eight centimeters dilated." Less than three hours later, her daughter was born.

WHO'S ON CALL?

If your midwife works alone, she is the one who will normally be with you for labor and delivery. Most group practices and birth centers have on-call systems for labor and delivery, with nurse-midwives working shifts of twelve or twenty-four hours, or for the weekend. Large hospital services and Health Maintenance Organizations have someone on duty in the hospital at all times. So you may not end up with "your" nurse-midwife for the birth, but it will probably be someone you saw for at least one prenatal visit, someone who will adhere to the philosophy and procedures you have been prepared to expect.

Rotating the on-call shift helps to make the midwife at your birth well-rested and focused on you. Audrey, who was a medical resident herself in an Ann Arbor hospital when she gave birth with nurse-midwives, knew first-hand what a resident's schedule was like. She liked knowing that her nurse-midwife would be relatively fresh, patient and focused solely on her: "Because Terri's practice works in shifts you don't run into the problem where your doctor was up all night the night before, and it looks like she's going to be up all night tonight, so she wants to hurry you up with Pitocin or do a cesarean so she can get to sleep."

In some HMOs and hospital birthing services, nurse-midwives assist two or three births during a twelve-hour shift. Most private practices, regardless of the birth setting, maintain a small enough midwife-to-mother ratio to practically assure one-on-one attention for a woman in active labor.

FIRST STAGE—ACTIVE LABOR

Toward the end of your pregnancy, your midwife encourages you to shape your own birth environment. You will be allowed to wear what you'd like, have relatives or friends present, and pick music that may help you relax during labor. Your midwife probably will even suggest that family members prepare food and drink while you are in labor for a birthday celebration afterward!

When it is time for you to go to the hospital or birth center, your nurse-midwife will usually meet you there. Typically, she examines your cervix to determine how far dilated you are, listens to the baby's heartbeat using a fetal stethoscope, or fetoscope and she, or a nurse, checks your blood pressure. They may also help you into the clothing you chose for the birth. From then on, your nurse-midwife remains with you throughout your labor.

She may encourage you to walk—a generally practical and productive alternative to lying in bed. Activity and simple gravity speed the baby toward the birth canal, applying pressure to the cervix so that it opens. Your midwife may walk with you, supporting you if you need it when a contraction comes. A nurse-midwife at Jackson Memorial Hospital in Miami "does the bump" with her patients: "You know, do a little boogey to help the baby out," she says. Nurse-midwives find that lying flat on your back in bed is perhaps the worst position for labor. Not only do you lose the effect of gravity, the position also can constrict a major artery that pumps blood toward the baby, which could contribute to fetal distress.

A nurse-midwife encourages you to try different positions throughout labor, to find what is most comfortable to cope with contractions. Lying on your side, bracing yourself on hands and knees, sitting upright or even on a toilet, are common positions, as is squatting, alone or with assistance from partner or midwife. This is a position most

North American women do not automatically think of, but it is wonderfully effective for labor. In a hospital bed or birthing chair, you can be propped to a 45-degree angle. Sitting up in a regular bed, supported by pillows or with your partner behind you works well, too. Nurse-midwives often recommend a shower, or a few minutes in a whirlpool tub if one is available. The pounding water can relieve tension and soothe pain so well that many women don't want to come out!

The optimal position for you may change as labor progresses. What works for one person may not be right for another. Not everyone feels good being in bed. Not everybody feels good walking or standing in the shower. If you are doing what feels good to you and making normal progress, a nurse-midwife will not interfere. If your progress slows, she may suggest getting out of bed to walk, or going into the shower.

Women find it a huge reassurance as labor takes over to have someone with an experienced eye alongside them who can say with authority that all is going just as nature planned. If you want the midwife out of your way, she steers clear. If you want her massaging your back, she is there. She makes sure you have ice chips or sips of juice and may suggest a heating pad for your belly or show your partner how to massage your lower back. If you want another pair of hands, she is there. The simple presence of a nurse-midwife can be an enormous comfort and help during those bewildering moments as contractions come closer and harder.

"Women can work themselves up to a point that they cannot cope with labor," said Marilynn Wender, a private practice nurse-midwife in Palm Beach County, Florida. "We try not to let the laboring woman get to that point. We act before the patient gets exhausted."

Most midwives make pain medication available and are qualified to administer those such as the analgesic Demerol, which may be offered when a woman seems overcome by labor or unable to cope with contractions. Nurse-midwives can also give Pitocin, which induces contractions and later helps control postpartum bleeding. In hospital births, they also can arrange for an anesthesiologist to administer an epidural, which numbs a woman from belly to knees. These and other drugs are used more frequently in hospital births.

PATIENCE

Sometimes labor, especially with a first baby, stretches for hours or even days from start to finish. A nurse-midwife will not rush in with labor-inducing drugs or a cesarean section. In hospital parlance "failure to progress" is the most frequent reason for a cesarean birth; but a nurse-midwife does not automatically classify a slow labor as a faulty one. If labor is not proceeding at textbook pace, a midwife is taught to consider a number of factors: she may gauge the health of the baby through its heartbeat and may take a sample of the fetal scalp blood to make sure enough oxygen is reaching the baby. She also considers the mother's stamina. If all seems fine, she allows nature to take its course.

Audrey, the Ann Arbor physician whose two sons were born in a hospital with nurse-midwives, spent fifty hours in labor with her first son. She stayed home for the first twenty-four hours and feels certain a doctor would have intervened with a cesarean or used forceps to help the baby out—procedures she very much wanted to avoid. In the end, she needed neither, in large part due to the nurse-midwife's approach.

When the baby's heart rate started to go down somewhat, rather than call for a cesarean, the nurse-midwife took a sample of the baby's fetal scalp blood. This showed that the baby was receiving adequate oxygen. She let Audrey proceed at her own pace.

"I pushed for four hours," Audrey said. "Obstetricians don't linger for four hours. They usually set it at two hours. It's not an absolute protocol, but usually if pushing goes on for more than two hours, then they use forceps."

Certainly the labor was exhausting, but in the end, she had a healthy son, a rapid recovery, and none of the procedures she had hoped to avoid.

That willingness to work one-on-one with a woman is a hallmark of nurse-midwives. Nurse-midwife Leslie Stewart now attends home births, but she remembers the contrast between her approach and the doctors' when she worked in a large, busy hospital in southern California. Often, doctors would order a cesarean section for "failure to progress," only to find that all operating rooms were full. Leslie would be asked to work with the woman in the meantime.

Leslie would help the woman out of bed and walk the halls with her, or encourage her to squat. Many times, the labor picked right up, and the woman delivered vaginally. The problem, Leslie said, is that a woman who is lying flat on her back often gets stalled in labor, and then discouraged.

A relaxed mother is also one of labor's best motivators. Nurse-midwife LaRita Evans has seen how anxiety can inhibit an otherwise normal labor. Many women come to labor very frightened, she says, and something as simple as a midwife's quiet presence can lend reassurance. LaRita's equipment for labor includes her knitting bag, which she brings to the hospital birthing room.

"I don't always knit a lot, but I always bring it," she said. "No matter how active their labor is, women always come up and ask me what I'm knitting. That kind of gets me in there. . . . Even if I am only able to do a few stitches it helps the mother and father feel that I am calm as we wait."

In a slow labor, a nurse-midwife might use a pause to ask if there is something the mother is concerned about, or afraid of. Many women harbor fears of a birth defect or not being able to push the baby out. Voicing those very real concerns, and hearing a midwife's reassurance, often is enough to free up a mother's energy so she can concentrate on the job at hand.

"I had a woman who already had a retarded child, and when she was in labor with the next child, she wouldn't push out that baby," LaRita said. "I said, 'You're not letting that baby out because you're afraid.' And she said, 'Yes, I'm afraid it will be retarded.' " Having spoken her fears, the woman gave birth to a normal and healthy child.

LaRita's goal is simply to help a laboring woman feel calm. "I sit there a long time, sometimes I just sit there on the couch," she said. "I pick up the knitting and the labor just gets going. I think it makes a big difference."

RECOGNIZING PROBLEMS—MEDICAL INTERVENTION

In a hospital, birth center, or home, a midwife's frequent checks and her familiarity with the woman keep her attuned to what is going on in the labor. Because she spends so much time with a woman, she is often able to detect the subtleties that indicate a problem very early, and head off that problem before it escalates.

If a labor begins to deviate from the normal, a nurse-midwife uses the least invasive measure first to get it back on track. Because she may detect a problem early she may not need to resort to a drastic corrective measure immediately. The art of midwifery includes many tricks—proven by experience, but not necessarily in textbooks—to quickly correct a faltering labor: if the baby's heart slows down, she helps the mother onto her left side to increase blood flow to the baby; or if labor slows, a warm bath to relax the mother. Efforts like these can help bring about a safe vaginal birth.

If a complication develops that falls outside the scope of normal birth, however, a nurse-midwife calls on her consulting physician. Depending on the situation, the obstetrician may take over the care, or simply advise the nurse-midwife how to proceed. Once the doctor is called in, his or her decision holds sway. This is true whether the setting is a hospital, birth center, or home. Good rapport between nurse-midwife and doctor is important at this point. In the best situations the two professionals work as a team, with the doctor giving weight to the midwife's perspective and the mother's wishes.

TRANSITION

If all proceeds normally, the first stage of labor culminates with very strong contractions close together. These few minutes—called "transition" because they mark the passage from the first stage of labor to the second—can be the most trying part of labor. A nurse-midwife is a particular comfort at this time when some women become frightened and nearly incoherent, unable to regain composure between contractions. A nurse-midwife encourages them to let go and not try to control the force that is driving through them. Their trust in her makes that easier to do.

When Roi began transition, she felt out of control, something alien to her calm and composed nature. Her natural instinct was to maintain decorum, to stay in control. But her midwife, with whom she was so comfortable, was able to move Roi beyond her inhibitions to work with the labor. Roi wanted to have a birth with as little medical intervention as possible, and the midwife helped her do it.

"It was very comforting for me that she was there," Roi said. "She kept saying things to me, like 'Don't worry, this is exactly what should be happening, you're doing fine.' I felt out of control. I had no medication, which is what I hoped for all along, although at one point I asked her if it was too late for drugs. She laughed and said it was!"

That's when Roi knew she was almost there.

SECOND STAGE—PUSHING AT LAST

For many women, transition ends with a lull, a few minutes to regain composure before contractions begin again. When they do, they usually bring with them an undeniable urge, at last, to push! Partners, prepared by childbirth education classes, are especially helpful at this point, supporting the woman in bed or in a squat position as she bears down with each contraction.

The midwife gives near-constant, positive encouragement through these last difficult hours of labor. It is extremely painful for many women as the baby's head moves through the bony structure of the pelvis. The pushing stage can last an hour or two, or more, for a first baby; it is usually less than an hour for subsequent children.

Your midwife knows the most comfortable way to adjust wherever your baby is, and will continue recommending different positions for you. If you are having back labor, for instance, she may suggest you try getting on hands and knees to relieve the pressure on your spine. Some birth centers have birthing stools—low-sitting stools, with boomerang-shaped seats—and some midwives bring them along to home and hospital births. The woman rests on the seat, or her partner sits there, and she leans against him.

A nurse-midwife remains a guide and coach. You may be concentrating so hard that you may forget momentarily what all the work is for, but the midwife keeps you focused on the reward almost at hand, turning the negative aspect of pain into positive thoughts of the baby it will bring. When your baby finally crowns, meaning the top of the head is visible, your midwife may position a mirror so you can see. She may guide your hand toward the first touch of your child—the perfect incentive for those last few pushes!

Meanwhile, the midwife is hard at work, continuing to monitor contractions and fetal heart rate. She also may massage the perineum to avoid an episiotomy. That incision, from the vagina toward the rectum, is made almost routinely by some doctors to facilitate birth. Like many mothers, Roi appreciated the efforts of her nurse-midwife to successfully avoid an episiotomy.

"She did a lot of massage and stretching of the perineum while I was in labor, with oils and things," Roi said. "I had a slight abrasion, but I didn't need stitches. I attribute a lot of that to Barbara. She worked very hard."

BIRTH

As the baby's head is born, the nurse-midwife helps it gently over the perineum, then guides the typical rotation of the tiny body as it slides out of the birth canal. The midwife may move to the side, so the father can take over and be the first to hold his own baby. Sometimes a mother reaches down to catch the baby herself, guided by instinct as she lifts the wet and crying newborn right onto her breast.

THIRD STAGE AND BEYOND

Many mothers are so excited once the baby arrives they barely notice labor's third stage, the delivery of the placenta. After the baby has let out its first cry, the midwife may offer the job of clamping and cutting the umbilical cord to the father or other family member. If there are no takers, she does it herself. A midwife may remind the distracted mother to push the placenta out with the last few contractions. Again, a nurse-midwife is patient, allowing a little more time for the placenta to be expelled naturally—very rarely does she remove it manually from the womb. A midwife's professional standard is to examine the placenta to make sure all of it has been expelled and to look for defects that could indicate inadequate nourishment to the fetus.

Nurse-midwives believe that a baby belongs to its parents and should remain with them. Cleaning, tests, and the eye ointment required in most states are usually administered in front of you, on or alongside your bed. The midwife often stays close by to observe mother and baby for at least an hour after the birth. She may massage your uterus to encourage contractions that will stop blood flow, and give Pitocin if necessary to help the uterus contract. She also signs the birth certificate.

A nurse-midwife usually encourages breastfeeding almost immediately after birth. Breastfeeding not only helps the uterus to contract but also encourages an early bond between you and your child. Some women find breastfeeding awkward at first, so the midwife often remains to assist. She proves that indeed this is something your clever infant already knows how to do quite well!

LAURA'S STORY

It was the nurse-midwife philosophy that attracted Laura. From books and friends, she developed the opinion that birth wasn't something that had to be *done* to a woman; it was something a woman does herself. Soon after she became pregnant, Laura attended the nurse-midwives' orientation at a hospital in her New York City neighborhood, and she liked what she heard.

"They said you can give birth in any position you want, standing up, sitting down, lying down, on all fours, in the bathroom, whatever you are comfortable with," she said. "That made me feel comfortable, because I didn't want it to be like an operation. They made me feel like the birth was something I would be in control of, and whatever felt good for me I could do. They were there to *help* deliver the baby, not to give orders."

A year earlier, she assisted at a friend's delivery and was bothered by what seemed like an angry tone from the doctors and nurses, "giving orders and sounding very uptight," she said. That was the last thing she wanted for her own labor.

"I didn't want someone yelling at me saying, 'You're doing it wrong,' or 'I told you to breathe,' " she said. "I knew I'd just break down and cry."

From the start, Laura was delighted with the care of her nurse-midwives. For the birth, she planned for her mother and sister to be at the hospital along with her husband, and their midwife.

When Laura arrived at the hospital after six hours of labor at home, she had no idea just how close she was to giving birth. According to all the books, a first-time mother still had hours to go, but by the time she and her husband reached the hospital admitting desk, the contractions were almost nonstop. She moaned through admitting, had contractions in the elevator and cried as she walked toward her room, grabbing the railing for support.

When she got to her room, her midwife and mother and sister were there. It was exactly the cheerful scene Laura had hoped for, but at that moment, nothing but the next contraction seemed to matter.

"You're allowed to bring your own nightgown, but by that point, I didn't care," she said. "I'd wear a sheet. I couldn't wait to get into bed."

The midwife's vaginal exam showed that Laura was dilated eight centimeters, a wonderful surprise for the first-time mother, who dreaded she was only three or four. No wonder she was feeling so crazy—she probably passed transition on the way to her room! The midwife placed the beltlike electronic fetal monitor across Laura's belly. Twenty minutes later, the contractions slowed down, so Laura got out of bed to walk.

"I stood up and walked around in two circles and then I was ready to push," she said. Her midwife lightly punctured her bag of waters with a long thin needle.

"I trusted her. If she felt I needed my waters broken, that was fine," Laura said. "It didn't hurt or anything. I didn't feel it."

Then came the hard work. After the first push, Laura thought, "This is painful!" Her goal was to push three times with each contraction. She began to get the sinking feeling that maybe it would be just too tough for her.

Then came the perfect inspiration.

"The longer and harder you push, the sooner you will have your baby," her nurse-midwife said.

That was all Laura needed to hear.

"When she said that, I thought, 'I am getting this kid out. I am going to push as long and hard as this contraction,' " Laura said. The baby's head crowned. A few more fierce pushes and 8-pound, 1-ounce Kaitlin was born.

Of course, not every new mother has the reaction she

has always dreamed of. When they handed Laura her baby, her first thought was, "Why are they doing this to me after what I've just been through? Give her to my husband!"

The baby looked so different from the child she had pictured, and that surprised her. Soon enough Laura, a blond, was laughing with delight over little Kaitlin's full head of brown hair. And she was very glad that her daughter was born into a calm and joyful setting.

"What was really nice about my birth is that everybody was so happy. The midwife was really nice, she never yelled at me, she always spoke very calmly," Laura said. "I'm not a hysterical person to begin with, I like just to be calm and in control. The midwife was nice and calm during the whole thing. That was important to me."

4.

ONLY WHEN NEEDED:

Medical Technology
and Nurse-Midwifery

*"People think that once you go to a midwife, you
are turning your back on technology. You're not
turning your back on it, you're maintaining it as
an alternative, not something that's automatic."*
—*LYDIA, A FIRST-TIME MOTHER*

LYDIA CHOSE TO HAVE her baby at home and needed virtually no medical intervention. As long as everything
proceeded normally and she felt confident, there was no
reason for an intravenous drip, drugs, or an episiotomy
and stitches, procedures standard in most non-midwife
births. A nurse-midwife will use them too, if they are
necessary; but if there is no clear reason to use them, why
meddle with a process nature designed to work so well?

Some of the medical interventions often used in typical
obstetrical birth are high-tech methods designed to gauge
infant health, such as continuous electronic fetal monitors. Others, such as enema and pubic shave, became
standard partly for the convenience of the medical sys-

tem. By the early 1980s, the specter of medical malpractice lawsuits led to a new style of "defensive medicine" that used certain tests and technology routinely. Some procedures became automatic, although no one had proven their necessity, benefit, or true effect. Many obstetricians never see a birth in which labor's natural flow is not interrupted by at least one hospital procedure. Many complete their education without ever sitting alongside a woman for a full labor, learning its natural rhythms.

Some parents believe that more is better when it comes to having a baby, that each type of intervention makes birth safer. But medical technology may also heighten the image of a pregnant woman as an ill person—someone who needs things to be done to her. Unquestionably, medical intervention saves the lives of mothers and babies who have specific complications. If no complication exists, however, intervention may interrupt nature's engineering and timing for your particular labor. One procedure may lead to another, beginning a domino effect of medical interference in a birth that could proceed safely on its own.

Consider this scenario: a laboring woman lies on her back in bed. Although she is not dehydrated, an intravenous line drips sugar water into her veins. Although the baby's heartbeat sounds fine, a continuous electronic fetal monitor is strapped on. These devices keep the woman lying still, but without activity and gravity to stimulate the labor, her progress stalls. She receives a labor-inducing drug, which produces violent contractions, making a painkiller necessary. The drugs or anesthesia then impede the woman's ability to push, requiring forceps to pull the baby out and an episiotomy to make room for the forceps.

In a typical birth attended by a nurse-midwife, this chain of events would not be set in motion. A laboring woman is encouraged to walk to keep her labor moving along. If there are signs that medical intervention are needed—an intravenous line for a dehydrated mother or a fetal monitor if the baby's heartbeat seems erratic—a nurse midwife's professional standard is to use them. The use of medical intervention varies, depending on whether the birth is in a hospital, birth center, or home.

Nurse-midwives use technology when needed to learn something about the pregnancy they otherwise would not know. They use it when the benefits to mother and child outweigh the risks. This chapter explains interventions frequently used in pregnancy and childbirth and a nurse-midwife's approach to each.

PRENATAL TESTING

To test or not to test is a question frequently left up to parents, with the nurse-midwife explaining the risk, benefit, and potential result of each test and sometimes strongly recommending or even ordering a test if she thinks the findings would influence a decision about the pregnancy. This summary of the most common tests explains how and when a nurse-midwife would use each one:

Ultrasound

What it is: A small device emitting high frequency sound waves is passed over your belly. As the waves bounce off internal structures, they are fed into a machine that electronically creates a picture, called a sonogram, of the fetus and its surroundings.

What it tells: A sonogram indicates a fetus's gestational age based on size and whether the fetus is developing properly. It also shows the position of the fetus and placenta. Some parents choose to have a sonogram for the thrill of seeing the fetus, to learn its sex (not always accurately), or for assurance that the fetus appears normal.

Risks: There are no proven dangers of ultrasound, but some parents prefer not to expose the fetus to sound waves.

Who performs it: Although a few nurse-midwives perform ultrasound themselves, it usually is done by a sonographer and interpreted by a radiologist in a hospital or test center. A nurse-midwife may help interpret the results of the sonogram.

A nurse-midwife recommends it: To rule out ectopic pregnancy or some congenital abnormalities; to confirm the diagnosis of twins; or make sure the fetus is growing properly when weight gain is small. An ultrasound can show whether unexplained bleeding late in pregnancy is due to placenta implantation over the cervix, a condition that calls for a cesarean. Ultrasound also can help determine the gestational age of the fetus, and therefore due date, if a woman is unsure when she conceived. A midwife then knows whether the baby is likely to be fully developed if labor starts early and can consider induction of labor if the pregnancy goes on too long.

Amniocentesis and Chorionic Villi Sampling (Genetic Testing)

What it is: Amniocentesis and chorionic villi sampling detect genetic abnormalities in a developing fetus by analyzing cells gathered from the uterine cavity. In amniocentesis, usually done between the fourteenth and eighteenth weeks of pregnancy, amniotic fluid is withdrawn through a needle inserted in the woman's abdomen; three weeks later a cell culture reveals genetic makeup. Chorionic villi sampling (CVS), a relatively new procedure, is done at eight to twelve weeks. A narrow tube inserted through the cervix removes placental cells that contain the same genetic makeup as the fetus. The cells are cultured and results are available within a week. The cells also can be withdrawn through a needle inserted in the mother's abdomen.

What it tells: Amniocentesis can reveal malformation of the brain or spinal cord, known as neural tube defect; some hereditary diseases; Down's syndrome; and other genetic disorders. Chorionic villi sampling detects similar diseases and chromosomal abnormalities, but does not detect neural tube defect.

Risks: Each test carries a small risk of miscarriage and/or infection.

Who performs it: Nurse-midwives do not perform CVS or amniocentesis. CVS is done in a doctor's office. Amniocentesis is usually a hospital outpatient procedure, although some doctors may do it in their offices.

A nurse-midwife recommends it: If there is family history of birth defects or hereditary disease, or if parents are carriers of a genetic disease. The tests are also common among women in their midthirties and older, for whom there is an increased chance of having a baby with Down's syndrome. A midwife explains the merits and disadvantages of each test and helps parents decide whether to have it done; they also refer women to genetic counselors as needed.

Alpha Fetoprotein Screen

What it is: This test of the mother's blood between the fifteenth and eighteenth weeks measures a protein manufactured by the fetus.

What it tells: A high level of alpha fetoprotein may indicate a malformation of the brain or spinal cord or other congenital abnormalities. A low level may indicate chromosomal abnormalities, including Down's syndrome.

Risks: There are no known risks. The test must be done when the fetus is a precise age though, because the level of alpha fetoprotein changes during pregnancy. A test done too early can result in a false positive.

Who performs it: A nurse-midwife, doctor, or nurse draws the mother's blood in the office, and sends it to a lab.

A nurse-midwife recommends it: Many nurse-midwives offer the test routinely.

Non-stress Test

What it is: The mother is hooked up to a electronic fetal monitor, which measures the fetal heart rate.

What it tells: Toward the end of pregnancy, the heart rate of a healthy fetus speeds up following each fetal movement. During a twenty-minute period, a healthy fetus shows two such accelerations, each lasting at least fifteen seconds. Normal accelerations indicate that the fetus is healthy and receiving enough oxygen via the placenta.

Risks: There are no known risks.

Who performs it: A doctor or nurse-midwife in an office, clinic, or hospital where the electronic monitor is available.

A nurse-midwife recommends it: When a pregnancy goes beyond forty or forty-two weeks, a nurse-midwife may suggest a non-stress test to gauge whether the placenta and fetal environment are still able to sustain the fetus. If the accelerations are too few or too short, it may be a sign that the fetus is not receiving adequate oxygen. A nurse-midwife may then suggest inducing labor.

If you are uncertain about testing, a nurse-midwife helps you through the decision. She provides statistical information. She prompts you to clarify your views on abortion and on raising a child with a disability, so you can approach these difficult issues realistically and in a way that suits your beliefs. She may refer you to a genetic center for counseling.

Roi, a Brooklyn mother who had her first baby at age thirty-six, described her nurse-midwives' attitude toward testing as "very non-opinionated, very factual." Her initial impulse was to refrain from tests that were not absolutely necessary. But she still wanted to hear the pros and cons.

"They gave us all the information and all the statistics, and then left it up to us to decide," she said. Roi and her husband chose against genetic testing. But, twice she opted for a sonogram. The first, at six weeks, was to make sure the pregnancy was not ectopic (developing in a fallopian tube), as a previous pregnancy had been. The second, at six months, was because Roi got very large and her midwives suspected—falsely, it turned out!—twins.

"PREP"—SHAVING AND ENEMA

Being "prepped"—or prepared—for labor in some hospitals still means shaving a woman's pubic area and giving her an enema. The rationale for shaving, which became standard procedure soon after birth moved into hospitals, was that the hair harbored germs that could infect the baby. Shaving also gave doctors an unobstructed view of the perineum to perform an episiotomy. By the 1960s, women questioned shaving, which many found degrading as well as itchy and painful as hair grew back. Research eventually showed that tiny nicks from the razor introduced a new risk of infection to the mother,[1] and doctors realized that hair on a clean body harbored no germs. Nurse-midwives do not shave women. On a rare occasion, they may snip a few hairs or shave a small area as needed for visibility in repairing an episiotomy.

Enemas are given with the rationale that emptying the lower intestine makes more room for the baby and saves everyone the embarrassment and mess of stool being pushed out as the baby is born. Most women, however, prefer to avoid the discomfort and slight indignity of an enema. Women usually have loose stools early in labor— nature's way of preparing for what is ahead—so nurse-midwives rarely find an enema necessary. If a woman loses control of her bowels, the midwife simply whisks away the disposable pads or sheets beneath her and replaces them with fresh ones.

INDUCING LABOR

Labor begins when a woman's body produces oxytocin, the natural hormone that makes the uterus contract. Just what triggers production of oxytocin is unknown. A synthetic version of oxytocin, Pitocin, is used by doctors and some nurse-midwives to induce a late or stalled labor. With Pitocin—which is not available outside the hospital—continuous fetal monitoring is necessary to make sure the baby receives enough oxygen during the unnaturally strong contractions it sometimes causes.

Doctors in some hospitals use Pitocin if a laboring woman does not meet the maternity ward's definition of progress (usually, one centimeter dilation per hour). Many doctors also induce labor if a specified amount of time has passed (usually twelve or twenty-four hours) since the bag of waters has broken, or if a woman is more than two weeks past her due date.

Nurse-midwives, in contrast, have few time measurements by which things should happen. Many women have start-and-stop labors that eventually pick up at their own pace. As long as the baby's heart rate is fine and the mother is not exhausted, dehydrated, or showing signs of infection, there is little need to interfere. If labor stalls, a midwife encourages a woman to walk or change positions before resorting to Pitocin.

For a post-date labor, a nurse-midwife tries to spur labor with more moderate measures before using Pitocin. A rapid walk may be enough to get you started. Intercourse, if you and your partner feel like it, may help because seminal fluid contains prostaglandins that soften the cervix and start labor. An enema, castor oil, or a laxative also may prompt labor by stimulating the intestines. Another low-tech tactic is nipple stimulation, which triggers the release of oxytocin into the bloodstream; but some midwives recommend this only in the hospital, because of the strong and sudden contractions it may bring on.

When water breaks before labor begins, some nurse-midwives will induce labor within twelve hours. Others allow a full day or more for the labor to begin on its own, with instructions not to take a bath or have intercourse—activities that can introduce infection. You may be asked to take your temperature every four hours, to tell whether you are developing an infection or fever.

When nurse-midwife concludes that a mother or baby is at risk, induction of labor is the likely course. Severe hypertension at the end of pregnancy, for example, may be a reason to induce labor rather than risk the mother or baby's health by allowing the pregnancy to go on any longer than necessary. Labor also may be induced if a mother is more than two weeks overdue, and a non-stress test indicates that the placenta is no longer functioning effectively. If a labor is going on so long that a mother may be too exhausted to push the baby out, a midwife may suggest Pitocin, in very small amounts at first, to move the labor along so the mother will have enough energy left to push.

BREAKING WATERS, OR AMNIOTOMY

If labor is progressing, a nurse-midwife will not break your bag of waters simply because it has not broken on its own. If the labor is unusually slow, she may discuss with you breaking the waters to spur it along. Artificial rupturing of membranes, called amniotomy, is done with a crochet-like hook inserted painlessly through the dilated cervix to puncture the sac. If you are ready to push and the waters have not broken, a midwife may break them, as happened with Laura, whose birth was described in Chapter 3. On very rare occasions, a baby is born with the bag still intact. According to folklore, babies born "in the caul" are destined for a lifetime of good fortune!

INTRAVENOUS DRIP

Getting plenty of fluids during labor keeps up a woman's energy and helps her uterus work efficiently. Many hospitals automatically start an intravenous line that drips sugar water into a vein in the laboring woman's hand or arm. The drip is unnecessary, though, if she is allowed to sip liquids. Nurse-midwives rarely use intravenous lines automatically, but, instead, encourage laboring women to drink plenty of water and juice. If intravenous medication is necessary, the line can be started within seconds.

When labor proceeds normally, the line is more of a hindrance than a help. It keeps a woman in bed and prevents her from walking, unless she wants to drag the IV pole, in addition to coping with labor pains. If she doesn't like using a bedpan, she may not empty her bladder as often; and a baby pressing on a full bladder makes for more painful contractions. Using the toilet frequently, as midwives encourage, empties the bladder and also keeps a laboring woman moving.

Eating light foods and drinking liquids during early labor fortifies a woman for what is ahead. To stay hydrated throughout labor, water, fruit juice, or honey tea do the trick without limiting movement. These refreshers chase away the cotton-mouth feeling that women get, and the juices are energizing.

Many hospitals, however, prohibit eating and drinking during labor. This is to prevent a woman from aspirating her stomach contents while under general anesthesia if a cesarean is necessary. Ironically, prohibiting food or drink could make a cesarean more likely: a woman unable to eat or drink through a very long labor may have less energy by the end to push her baby out. A study of women who had cesareans after being transferred from a birth center to a hospital showed that of the 115 who ate solid food during labor, none aspirated stomach contents while under anesthesia.[2] Although most cesarean sections are done under regional anesthesia, most hospitals prohibit anything but ice chips. If general anesthesia is used, a tube can be inserted to minimize the risk of aspiration.

Although nurse-midwives do not use IV lines regularly, they are sometimes necessary: if a woman is getting dehydrated because she is too nauseated by labor to drink;

if she is exhausted by a long labor; to administer Pitocin; or if there is a likelihood of cesarean.

"It's not that we're opposed to using an IV," said a nurse-midwife who works in a large Detroit hospital. "You look at the indications and make a decision. If you have a normal, healthy woman in labor and the baby is doing fine, there's no indication at all."

FETAL MONITORING

Continuous electronic fetal monitoring was introduced in the 1970s, and quickly became standard in conventional obstetrics. More recent scrutiny has made it the subject of considerable debate. There are two types of electronic fetal monitors: external and internal. The external monitor, which can be used at any time during pregnancy and labor, consists of a double belt placed across a mother's belly. One belt gauges the baby's heart rate using soundwaves; the other measures the strength and frequency of contractions. An internal monitor, used only in labor because it requires the bag of waters to be broken, is inserted through the vagina. An electrode screwed lightly into the baby's scalp measures the fetal heart rate while another instrument gauges the contractions. Both types of monitors produce continual data that appear on an electronic screen and paper tracings called a "strip." In normal labor, the strip shows how the baby's heart rate responds to each contraction—speeding up and then stabilizing. Too much or too little heart activity could signify a problem.

Fetal monitors were integrated rapidly into standard obstetrical care, based on the commonsense assumption that they would warn of fetal distress in time to save the baby or thwart brain damage with quick delivery by forceps or cesarean. The monitors were developed as a research tool, but their introduction happened to come at a time of physicians' increasing concerns over malpractice liability. Doctors liked having a paper record of the fetal heartbeat that could be used in court to show whether there were signs of distress during labor.

The monitors became popular without clear evidence that they provided better results than the "old-fashioned" practice of checking a baby's heartbeat at regular intervals with a fetal stethoscope or a hand-held Doppler, which works by soundwaves and enables everyone in the room to hear the heartbeat. By the late 1980s, studies showed that electronic fetal monitoring did not reduce newborn death, and there was little evidence that the monitors reduced the risk of neurological disorders.[3] There was concern that false signals, caused by a mother's coughs or movements while wearing an external monitor, and erroneous interpretations were leading to unnecessary cesareans. In 1989, the American College of Obstetricians and Gynecologists advised its members that listening with a fetoscope or Doppler every fifteen minutes during the first stage of labor and every five minutes during the pushing stage was as beneficial as continuous electronic fetal monitoring, even for a woman at risk of complications. For low-risk women, a reading every thirty minutes during active labor and every fifteen minutes during the pushing stage was appropriate.[4]

Nurse-midwives have steered away from continuous electronic fetal monitoring if there is no indication for it, in favor of regular checks with a fetoscope. One reason is that a woman hooked to an electronic monitor cannot get out of bed readily. Another disconcerting result is that the machine with the screen seems to command more attention than the woman herself. Touching and listening to a woman provide valuable clues about the labor that may be lost if everyone focuses on the monitor.

"I find I do it myself—I walk into the room and watch the monitor," said a nurse-midwife at Hutzel Hospital in Detroit. "When the monitor is on, the focus is on the monitor and not on the patient, not on the person in labor. The support people are a lot more supportive if you don't have that to look at. You look at the woman."

Fetal monitors are rarely used in birth centers or home births. Nurse-midwives in hospitals use monitors for specific situations, such as an extreme change in the baby's heart rate or very high maternal blood pressure. Electronic monitoring is needed with Pitocin, to gauge how the baby is weathering the strong contractions. The presence of meconium, the baby's first bowel movement, in the amniotic fluid also may prompt use of a monitor because the meconium may indicate fetal distress. In some hospitals, midwives use the monitors off and on: fifteen or twenty minutes with the external monitor when a mother first arrives, followed by intermittent electronic monitoring throughout the labor.

SOMETHING FOR THE PAIN

Two types of pain relief are used in labor: analgesics and anesthetics. Analgesic drugs, including the commonly used narcotic Demerol, are given by intravenous line or injection in varying doses during the first stage of active labor. Some women find Demerol eases the pain of contractions; others find it mostly relaxes them enough to handle the contractions better and to doze in between.

General anesthesia produces unconsciousness; regional anesthesia, which is far more common in labor, numbs targeted parts of the body. The most frequently used regional anesthetic is the epidural, given by injection any time in active labor by a physician who specializes in anesthesiology. It generally numbs the woman between

the knees and the waist while she remains lucid, and it
can be given in repeated doses during labor and delivery.
Other regional anesthetics include the pudendal block,
which numbs the perineum for delivery; the paracervical
block, which numbs the cervix; and the spinal block, which
causes numbness from the waist down. Either an epidural, spinal, or general anesthesia can be used for cesarean delivery. A local anesthetic, which affects smaller areas,
is often given by injection or spray to the perineum prior
to stitching an episiotomy or tear.

The benefits of pain medication and anesthesia are ob-
vious, but there can be detrimental side effects that may
prompt further intervention. Analgesics make some
women too drowsy to participate much in the labor or to
push their baby out, requiring forceps or possibly cesarean section. Depending on the timing and the dose, the
narcotic may cross the placenta and temporarily impair
the baby's ability to breathe and suck. Epidurals are
thought by some women to be a magic shot for coping
with labor, but they also may slow labor and inhibit a
woman's ability to push, making delivery by forceps or
cesarean more likely. Occasionally, epidurals also cause a
sudden drop in maternal blood pressure. As anesthesia
wears off, some women get headaches and feel shaky.

Pain is an undeniable aspect of childbirth for most
women, but many who anticipate that reality find it manageable without drugs. Being relaxed, confident and well-
informed goes a long way in helping a woman cope. An
early advocate of natural childbirth, Dr. Grantly Dick-
Read of England, described labor as a potential cycle of
fear, which causes tension, resulting in more pain, which
feeds the fear. A nurse-midwife cannot completely control labor and delivery, but she can help alleviate that fear,
starting during the prenatal months. During labor she helps
control the risk factors, and reduces the anxiety response.

Human contact and reassurance are preferable to pain

medication to help you relax so you can go with the flow of what your body is trying to accomplish. Labor becomes more painful and traumatic if, consciously or not, you fight the contractions and resist the natural forces at work to birth your baby. No amount of reading or talking can fully prepare you for childbirth, but it can instill an attitude that will help you summon the strength to cope with labor. The goal is for you to be a full participant, without drugged side effects, in the miracle of birth.

Louise gave birth to three children in a birth center and one at home, each time without medication. She liked being fully involved with the births. Some women have the notion that childbirth should not involve pain, she said. But it does, and it is manageable.

"It even says it in the Bible," she said. "But we have a society where people don't think there should be pain. It comes and goes. It's not that bad."

Nurse-midwives view pain relief as they do other medical interventions in childbirth: wonderful when necessary, but not to be used automatically. Many women choose nurse-midwives specifically to avoid drugs. The type of pain relief available depends on the philosophy of your midwife and the place of birth. Some nurse-midwives in hospitals use epidurals for vaginal birth at a mother's request; others believe the risk outweighs the benefit. Neither general nor epidural anesthesia is available outside the hospital because it must be given by an anesthesiologist and can lead to complications. Analgesics are available in birth centers and at home births, but women in these settings are so relaxed and confident that they rarely feel a need for medication. Nurse-midwives who have women assigned to them use pain medication more frequently; those women expect more medical intervention and have not sought out the nurse-midwife approach for their birth.

In certain situations, some nurse-midwives suggest pain

relief. If a woman's very slow progress seems due to anxiety, an analgesic or a mild tranquilizer may relax her enough that contractions pick up without using Pitocin. If a very long labor is depleting a woman's energy, pain medication may enable her to rest between contractions.

When Denise, the hospital social worker from suburban Detroit, was giving birth to her second daughter in a hospital, her midwife sensed she was becoming thoroughly exhausted. Denise already had an intravenous line and the nurse-midwife suggested medication. Denise, who had hoped for an unmedicated birth, asked whether she would still be lucid and able to push with Demerol. Her nurse-midwife answered all her questions, and Denise decided that medication, at that point, was a good idea. A few hours later, she delivered a healthy girl with no complications.

"It was my choice," Denise said. "If I had said no, that would have been okay too. She made the recommendation because she could see I was having a little difficulty. She could have just plugged it into my IV without my knowledge, or she could have told me drugs were the worst thing in the world. She gave me just enough medication to take the edge off, and that made all the difference."

Denise appreciated her midwife's upfront attitude. Together they made a decision they agreed was the right one for mother and baby.

FORCEPS AND VACUUM EXTRACTION

Forceps are grasping instruments with spoon-shaped ends that are eased over a baby's head to help assist the baby through the birth canal. Very few nurse-midwives use them. If forceps seem necessary for a long pushing stage or posterior baby, a nurse-midwife almost always calls the consulting physician. On very rare occasions, nurse-midwives use vacuum extraction. This involves placing on the baby's head a small cap attached to a machine that uses gentle suction to help the baby out.

CESAREAN BIRTH

Cesarean birth involves anesthetizing the mother and cutting through her abdomen and uterus to remove the baby. The baby is delivered within the first few minutes; it takes about forty minutes more to suture the tissues closed. By the late 1980s, 25 percent of births in the U.S. were by cesarean section, a sharp increase from 5 percent during the late 1960s. A major factor in this increase was doctors' concern over malpractice suits. Presented with even the slightest doubt as to whether a baby was receiving adequate oxygen, some doctors and hospitals opted for a cesarean, rather than run the risk of accusation later that a baby was impaired because a physician failed to act on signals of fetal distress. A trend of lawsuits, huge jury awards to families, and rising malpractice insurance premiums contributed to this type of defensive medicine. The use of fetal monitors, and perhaps their misreading, may have also contributed to the cesarean increase.

Cesareans are clearly called for when vaginal delivery could be dangerous for mother or baby due to placenta implantation over the cervix, a mother's chronic disease, a baby too big for the mother's pelvis, or a post-date baby seemingly unable to withstand an induced vaginal delivery. Other cesarean deliveries are done in response to an emergency in labor—if a baby's heart rate suddenly plummets, for example.

Cesarean birth is the most extreme intervention: it is major abdominal surgery that can bring a host of complications as well as the side effects of anesthesia, a more difficult recuperation, and a longer hospital stay than vaginal birth. It also deprives a mother of the powerful feeling of giving birth to her child. And it is more expensive.

Vaginal delivery, with minimal intervention, allows a mother to enjoy her baby right away. It also has built-in benefits for the infant: the tight squeeze through the mother's birth canal compresses the baby's chest, forcing it to expel fluid from its lungs as it moves toward the vaginal opening. This makes the baby's breathing easier during the first moments outside the womb, and may minimize respiratory problems later. The baby's head sometimes becomes elongated, or "molded," during a tight passage through its mother's pelvis, but it quickly returns to a more attractive, rounded shape with no damage.

Statistics show you are far less likely to have a cesarean birth if you have your baby with a nurse-midwife. CNMs do not perform the procedure, but call upon a physician when they determine that a vaginal birth would be risky for mother or child. Nurse-midwives maintain a cesarean rate of about 5 to 10 percent, compared to the overall U.S. rate of nearly 25 percent. For instance, at Women's Health Associates, Inc., a private practice of doctors and nurse-midwives outside Boston, 7.9 percent of 2,400 births were cesarean. In 1990 at Midwifery Services, Inc., in New York, 9.6 percent of 146 hospital births were cesarean. At The Women's Center of Martin County, a South Florida birth center, 5.5 percent of 237 women had cesareans. Home Birth Service of Los Angeles had a 2.9 percent cesarean rate for 700 women who began labor at home from 1984 through 1989.

The fact that nurse-midwives accept those women at low medical risk who are less likely to need cesareans partially explains their low rate of surgical birth. More importantly, nurse-midwives try to keep the pregnancy and labor as normal as possible, so that they can avoid medical interference that could lead to a cesarean. Prior to labor, a midwife never assumes that a cesarean will be necessary because of a woman's attitude; prenatal education and reassurance can change that outlook by the time of birth. A mother's small pelvis is also no reason to assume a cesarean will be necessary; if a woman is petite, she will likely grow a small baby.

If it becomes apparent during prenatal care with a nurse-midwife that you will need a cesarean, you will probably transfer to a doctor's care. Reasons could include severe gestational diabetes or a fetus positioned crosswise in the uterus. Depending on the doctor-midwife relationships and hospital rules, a midwife may co-manage prenatal care with the doctor and remain with you throughout the operation. The same may be true when a problem during labor, such as a detached placenta or the delivery of the umbilical cord before the baby, requires an emergency cesarean.

Many women choose nurse-midwives specifically to reduce their chances of a cesarean birth. To Audrey, the Ann Arbor doctor whose sons were delivered by nurse-midwives in a hospital, it made sense to do whatever she could to minimize the likelihood of surgery.

"I do not want to get cut open," she said. "I'm going to go with who has the lowest cesarean statistics. I figure if I have to, I have to, but I don't want a cesarean unnecessarily."

VAGINAL BIRTH AFTER A CESAREAN

"Once a cesarean, always a cesarean" was a long-time obstetrical credo. It was believed that once an incision was made to a woman's uterus, the strain of a subsequent attempt at vaginal delivery would rupture the scar. Many people also assumed that whatever complication required the first cesarean would occur again with the next baby.

Gradually, though, both notions are being proven wrong. Scar tissue is able to withstand labor, and the horizontal incisions to the uterus used in recent years are less likely to rupture than the vertical incisions they replaced. It is also acknowledged now that each birth is different. Even though a first baby was breech and needed a cesarean, a younger sibling may line up in perfect head-down position for labor.

Vaginal birth after cesarean (VBAC) has become increasingly common. In 1988, the American College of Obstetricians and Gynecologists (ACOG) recommended that women with one previous cesarean, with a low transverse incision, should be encouraged to attempt labor and vaginal delivery. ACOG cited studies showing that more than half of all women with low transverse incisions for a previous birth were successful at vaginal birth in a subsequent pregnancy, with a lower mortality rate for both mother and infant than with repeat cesareans.[5]

Most, but not all, nurse-midwives accept women who have had a prior cesarean birth and want to try vaginal delivery. Although VBACs clearly are possible and safe, some birth centers and home birth midwives feel they should be done only in a hospital. In some cases, whether a nurse-midwife accepts women for VBACs is determined by the doctors and administrators where she works. For women who would like to try VBAC, nurse-midwives are wonderful at providing the extra encouragement they may need if a prior cesarean left them less than confident in their body's ability to give birth.

EPISIOTOMY

This small cut in a laboring woman's perineal tissue is made with surgical scissors during the final moments of labor to allow quicker delivery of the baby's head. The rationale for an episiotomy has been to diminish trauma to the baby as it pushed against the perineal tissue and to prevent the tissue from tearing uncontrollably. But studies show that slow delivery of the head over an intact perineum does not compromise the newborn's health.[6] A small tear is no more likely to extend to the rectum than an episiotomy is.

An episiotomy requires stitches, which may be painful and itchy during the few weeks it takes for the cut and suturing to heal. Some women also find an episiotomy delays resumption of sexual relations, which may be painful until healing is complete. For these reasons, most women prefer to avoid an episiotomy, although many do not realize this is possible.

Nurse-midwives are skilled at making the scissor cut, but find it unnecesssary in the majority of births. They show women how to massage the perineum prior to labor to help stretch the tissue. During labor and delivery, a nurse-midwife works with mother and baby so that the head, usually the widest part of the baby, can be delivered slowly without a cut. Midwives place warm compresses on the perineum to relax the tissue and make it more flexible, or massage and stretch it with warm oil. In addition, a midwife does not routinely have a woman deliver in the traditional lithotomy position, on her back with legs up in stirrups. Women delivering with nurse-midwives give birth in whatever position is most comfortable—sitting, lying knees to chest, lying on one side—all of which better accommodate the baby.

A nurse-midwife's gentle-birth approach for a slow delivery means she coaches the woman through a few extra pushes as she guides the baby over the perineum. The results: many women end up with nothing more than a slight abrasion, or "skidmark," that heals quickly without stitches. A small tear generally is preferable to a cut, because it requires fewer stitches and less healing time and generally does not extend into the vaginal muscles, as an episiotomy does.

An episiotomy may be called for, though, if the baby is in distress and must be delivered quickly, or if it is clear that the mother will have a large tear. Nurse-midwives try to make the snip no larger than necessary. Nurse-midwives happily report that some doctors are no longer doing episiotomies routinely, having observed in midwife births that it may not be necessary.

SKIN-TO-SKIN

THERE IS NO better warming device for a new baby than the labor-warm body of its mother. The ideal place for a newborn is touching skin-to-skin on its mother's belly or breast. Babies traditionally have been born into delivery rooms that are kept cool, for the comfort of personnel and for safety near volatile anesthesia gases. The baby is then whisked into a criblike infant warmer or wrapped up mummylike for parents to hold. Most nurse-midwife births, in contrast, occur in a warm birthing room. The newborn immediately is cuddled by its parents, with its first sensations outside the womb likely to be a mother's warm breast and a father's caress.

A 1980 study in the *Journal of Nurse-Midwifery* compared body temperatures of babies placed in an infant warmer with those held skin-to-skin by their mothers. Of 51 babies, those who had only skin-to-skin contact during the first 45 minutes after birth maintained higher body temperatures than babies in warmers or babies who had a few minutes of each. The babies most likely to have below-normal temperatures either 21 or 45 minutes after birth were those who went right into a warmer, with no skin-to-skin contact.[7]

POST-BIRTH PITOCIN

In many hospitals, Pitocin is given automatically by intravenous or by injection after birth to help the uterus contract, which controls postpartum bleeding. Many nurse-midwives do not use the synthetic hormone automatically, preferring to see whether it will be necessary. Instead they encourage immediate breastfeeding, which stimulates natural production of oxytocin, the hormone that Pitocin mimics. Many mothers who nurse right after birth produce enough of the hormone to control most of the bleeding without drugs, although a small amount of bleeding in subsequent days is normal.

THE ART AND CRAFT OF NURSE-MIDWIFERY

Throughout pregnancy and labor, a nurse-midwife is full of tips for coping with the changes your body is undergoing. Most of these remedies and soothers could not be found in a medical textbook. But midwives know from experience that certain remedies work, be it ginger root to curb morning sickness, ice to numb painful breasts during the first weeks of nursing, or putting a laboring woman on her hands and knees if the baby's shoulder is slow to deliver.

Jane, the New York lawyer who went on a business trip during her eighth month, cherished the knowledge and experience of her nurse-midwives when it came to helping her through the minor discomforts of pregnancy. When she developed an intolerable (not to mention embarrassing) itch on her belly, her nurse-midwife knew the itch was caused by the stretching of her skin and it was not a major medical problem. She also knew it was driving Jane nuts, making pregnancy nearly unbearable for a while. She recommended vitamin E oil, rubbed directly into the skin. It worked. When Jane developed leg cramps, vitamin E again was suggested, this time by ingestion. That worked too.

Jane wanted pregnancy to disrupt her life as little as possible, and she was delighted with the relief these remedies gave her. But when her hay fever acted up and nothing the midwives suggested helped, they recommended she see an ear, nose, and throat specialist. The doctor's prescriptions relieved her symptoms.

"What I liked was that the midwives were willing to try different things," Jane said. "When something wasn't working, they didn't insist that you should try only natural remedies, and they didn't say 'suffer it out, blow your nose, think good thoughts and you'll get through.' They said, 'If you are suffering so miserably that it is going to worsen your pregnancy, get yourself to a doctor.' "

Throughout pregnancy and labor, a nurse-midwife uses whatever modern technology has to offer—but she does not do so automatically. From the start, she helps you make decisions based on what is going on with *your* pregnancy.

For this personal, low-tech care to work best, it is important that you and your nurse-midwife share a common outlook. You will be making decisions that involve weighing the pros and cons of technical intervention in childbirth. Nurse-midwives believe that their approach is the safest as well as most satisfying way to have a baby, but when it comes to your baby, the decisions are yours—for a lifetime.

"When there's a bad outcome and every available technology was used, people look back and say, 'Well we did everything we could,' " nurse-midwife Lisa Summers said. "Even though 'everything we could' may not have helped in the long run, and may have even added to a problem. But if you don't use all of that, you may look back and say, 'Gee, if I only had used a monitor, if I only had an IV.'

"It takes a tremendous amount of courage in this day and age to be with women in labor and to have faith and depend on the normalcy of birth rather than on IVs and monitors and operating rooms."

With hands of flesh, not contraptions of steel, is the way a nurse-midwife approaches pregnancy, and it is important for you to be comfortable with that. Learning about what happens during pregnancy and childbirth is the best way for you to make educated choices that are in sync with your personal values. A nurse-midwife birth experience may not be best for everyone. The next chapter will help you decide whether it is right for you.

5.

MOM AND MIDWIFE:
___

Is This the
Match for You?

"Whoever you see, you're going to see for nine months. You're really going to be intimate. And you obviously have to feel comfortable with that person in the end. Shopping for care is a process definitely worth doing."

—*DENISE*

"So much of having a good experience relates to your state of mind. You have to be comfortable. If you feel confident and positive, it just affects the whole experience."

—*ROI*

"It's a people thing. We're buying people. We're buying judgment. We're buying reaction, as consumers. That's the most important thing to us. Who's going to be with us and do we trust their judgment? At the moment when our knowledge

*runs out or our emotional circuits get overloaded,
do we trust a judgment call that's going to be
made by the person we're with?"*
        —DANIEL, JANE'S HUSBAND

YOU LIST YOUR priorities and comparison shop for a new
car, home, or even a microwave oven. Shouldn't you do
at least as much for something as precious as the well-
being of you and your baby? Denise, Roi, and Jane all
thought so, and that is why they chose nurse-midwives.
They found someone who shared their outlook on pregnancy and childbirth, someone whom they liked personally. They each created the ideal situation, one that fos-
tered the trust and emotional support that is crucial in
childbirth.

Not every woman is suitable for nurse-midwife care,
however. Medically, certain conditions may disqualify you.
Emotionally and intellectually, being comfortable with the
notion of nurse-midwifery is equally important. The goal
is for you to be with a health-care provider who makes
you feel confident and relaxed. There is no need for anxiety to sap your energy at a time when you need it most.
Your health-care choice should empower you to have a
positive and healthy experience.

This chapter poses questions to ask both doctors and
nurse-midwives as you weigh your options, and explains
some medical conditions that could disqualify you from
care with a nurse-midwife. It also lists questions to ask
yourself, as you decide whether you are temperamentally
and medically suited to having your baby with a nurse-
midwife.

DO YOU QUALIFY, MEDICALLY, AT THE START?

A nurse-midwife is a specialist in normal pregnancy and
birth. She does not want to jeopardize your health and

her professional standing by taking on a pregnancy that has a risk of complication outside her area of expertise. If you have a chronic condition that could complicate your pregnancy, you likely will not be accepted for nurse-midwifery care. Such conditions include: heart, lung, or kidney disease; organ transplant; insulin-dependent diabetes; severe hypertension; psychiatric illness that requires medication. Other conditions in some situations include obesity or below-normal weight, heavy drinking or use of illegal drugs. Sometimes smokers are not accepted for out-of-hospital births.

However, pregnancy may be carried out successfully by women with most of these conditions. Obstetricians go through years of training to care for just such high-risk pregnancies in which an existing medical condition may complicate, or be exacerbated by, pregnancy and childbirth.

Age is rarely considered a risk factor now. For years it was perceived that an "older" mother—from her mid-thirties on—was at greater risk during pregnancy and childbirth. Many people now find that good health is more important than age for safe childbearing. Most nurse-midwives have no age criteria, although some home birth practices and birth centers set a maximum age for first-time mothers.

The guidelines for whom a nurse-midwife accepts vary from one practice to the next, often depending on the place of birth and the arrangement with a doctor. Some conditions are considered borderline—acceptable for some midwife practices but not for others. Depending on their working relationship the doctor and nurse-midwife may co-manage a woman's care. Generally, a midwife who works in the same building with her consulting physician takes on a wider range of patients than a colleague whose office practice includes only nurse-midwives. In an HMO (Health Maintenance Organization), for instance, a nurse-midwife may accept a woman with a heart condition if it is controlled by medication. In public clinics or hospitals, nurse-midwives may include in their care women with chronic health problems. Midwife-only practices tend to be the most selective, especially if women in their care deliver in birth centers or at home.

PREGNANCY COMPLICATIONS THAT REQUIRE TRANSFER TO A DOCTOR

Even a pregnancy that starts off completely normal can develop complications. If this happens to you, and your heart is set on a natural birth with a nurse-midwife, you may feel horribly disappointed, even cheated. But nurse-midwifery's standard is to seek medical consultation for most complications. Whether you switch completely to a doctor again depends on your health status and the arrangement between your midwife and her consulting doctor.

Two of the most common medical problems during pregnancy are high blood pressure and gestational diabetes. In both cases, the mother usually returns to her pre-pregnancy good health after birth, but both can be serious during pregnancy, and require close supervision for the safety of both mother and child. In practices where a doctor and midwife work together, women with these conditions are likely to be co-managed: after a visit with a doctor you return to the care of your midwife, who is to keep the doctor informed of your status. In other practices, it may be necessary for you to switch completely to the physician's care.

Pregnancy-induced hypertension: About 7 percent of all pregnant women develop some form of elevated blood pressure, once called toxemia, which could put the fetus at risk of not receiving enough oxygen. In mild cases, known as pregnancy-induced hypertension, the woman is told to get extra rest and a doctor is generally consulted. If the situation is not extreme, a nurse-midwife may remain the caregiver. But if blood pressure rises dramatically or early in pregnancy, the physician will likely take over the woman's care. If blood pressure continues to rise and is accompanied by other signs, a condition known as pre-eclampsia, bed rest may be suggested. If this occurs near the end of pregnancy, as is most common, the nurse-midwife and physician may decide to induce labor.

Gestational diabetes: Gestational diabetes, an inability to metabolize sugar appropriately, is also frequently treated by a nurse-midwife or co-managed with her consulting physician. Once detected, it often can be controlled through diet and monitored with frequent blood tests. Some nurse-midwives refer women with gestational diabetes to doctors because the condition may engender other medical problems; others may keep a physician apprised of the woman's condition while monitoring her. A nutritionist may also be consulted. If gestational diabetes advances to the point that a pregnant woman must take insulin, she should go into the care of a physician.

Multiple births: When a pregnancy turns out to be twins, some nurse-midwives remain involved in the care; others refer the woman to an obstetrician. If a nurse-midwife participates in the delivery, it is with a physician present.

Breeches: Breech babies are not automatically transferred prenatally to a doctor for cesarean. Usually a midwife will give the baby time to flip into the head-first position. If the baby is transverse (lying sideways in the womb) near the end of pregnancy, it is standard to call in a doctor for a cesarean delivery. Other breeches are sometimes delivered vaginally.

Early and late babies: When labor begins before the 37th week of pregnancy, a nurse-midwife generally calls in the consulting physician. The same is true if a pregnancy continues beyond 42 weeks.

DO YOU QUALIFY EMOTIONALLY?

Sarah, who had three births with a nurse-midwife in a hospital in Palm Beach County, Florida, was stumped when asked to name any qualities other than medical condition that would make a woman unsuitable for midwifery care.

"I can't imagine anyone not having their pregnancy enhanced by a nurse-midwife," she said. "It's the most wonderful thing. It ought to be made a legal necessity. To me, the idea of doing it without a nurse-midwife is insane."

Sarah is a can-do type, willing and eager to take on responsibilities, important qualities if a woman is to thrive with a nurse-midwife. Although Sarah is right that a nurse-midwife probably would enhance the care of any pregnant woman, not all women are comfortable making that choice. If you have options in health care, you should seek care that addresses your needs. Your partner's concerns should also be included—after all, you are going through this together. Confront your own biases and realistically match your needs and beliefs with the person who will be caring for you. The following questions will help you assess whether a nurse-midwife is the right choice for you.

Do you believe in the ability of your body to give birth?

If you start out with the notion that birth is a natural, healthy process that your body knows how to do—with no prior experience or training!—you are right in line for nurse-midwife care. Confidence in the ability of your body to nurture and grow a fetus is an attitude that nurse-midwives cultivate in women. If you hold this belief at the start, you are on your way to having a positive experience.

Certainly most women have qualms about pregnancy: Will I stick to a good diet? Can my body actually carry out a birth? Women who have had cesarean births or miscarriages have more doubts than others about pregnancy in general and their own bodies in particular. But that does not mean their pregnancies cannot thrive and lead to healthy, safe vaginal births.

Any woman who qualifies medically and believes that a healthy, normal birth is part of nature's design for her is a good candidate for nurse-midwife care.

Are you willing to be an active participant in your own care with the decision-making responsibility that entails?

Even some women who are very assertive in other aspects of their life take a passive role when it comes to health care. There is room for a lot of personal decision-making in pregnancy and childbirth.

"If you want to be told what to do, it's silly to go to a midwife because it is interactive," said Daniel, who went to many of his wife's prenatal visits with nurse-midwife Barbara Brennan. "If you're not interacting, there's nothing happening."

That does not mean a nurse-midwife expects you to know the entire physiology and anatomy of birth at your first prenatal visit, or to be an expert by the end. She teaches the necessary specifics as the pregnancy goes along. Generally, though, the best candidates for midwife care

are those who are eager to learn about what is going on with their bodies and how they can contribute to the outcome. Childbirth can include so many choices—prenatal testing, who to have at the birth, how you will care for yourself during pregnancy. A midwife wants you to read, ask questions, and go to classes so you will be able to make informed decisions.

"Women have to be comfortable enough and secure enough within themselves to want to explore the various alternatives that are available to them," said Barbara Brennan, "and certainly have their partners participate."

What do you, your partner, and your midwife expect your partner's role to be?

A nurse-midwife expects you to have a support person with you during labor. This is usually the baby's father, but can also be your mother, sister, or friend. That person is expected to attend childbirth classes, learn about pregnancy, and attend at least one prenatal visit. This childbirth team of mother, partner, and midwife works best if all participants have the same expectations.

Most private practice nurse-midwives assume your partner will be involved in the pregnancy and labor. Some fathers simply are not comfortable with these roles, and that should be a factor in your decision-making. A little hesitation is normal; many fathers then surprise themselves by how quickly and naturally they overcome their reluctance as the pregnancy begins to seem more real. If someone has serious reservations or complete lack of interest, these concerns should be acknowledged and taken into account.

Because a nurse-midwife views pregnancy holistically, she knows that your partner's attitudes can have a strong impact on your emotional health during your pregnancy. If your partner is skeptical about nurse-midwife care, you may feel uneasy about making that choice. Doubts should be talked out early, perhaps with a midwife's help.

*Will you feel comfortable facing pregnancy and birth
without a doctor by your side?*

In the past two or three generations, birth has become so medicalized that some people find it hard to shake the bias that pregnancy is safe only in the hands of someone who has a medical degree. This may be especially true for you if there are doctors in your family or if you always have felt a bit of reverence for the medical profession. If you regard pregnancy and labor as medical conditions, not natural functions of your body, then you may have difficulty regarding nurse-midwife care as safe.

"People have the right to choose," said nurse-midwife Jan Kriebs, who works in a Washington, D.C., HMO. "If they are uncomfortable with the concept of me providing their care, I shouldn't be doing it."

The thousands of women who have their babies with nurse-midwives each year, however, find that the expertise, good judgment, and openness of a nurse-midwife provide the perfect approach to childbirth. Karen, who went to nurse-midwives for her second pregnancy more out of convenience than conviction, found the balance between nurse-midwife and doctor to be just right. "I didn't feel for an instant that the nurse-midwives couldn't answer one of my questions, or were not qualified to answer," she said. "And I felt that if *they* had a question, they would go to the doctor. The doctor was always in the background."

*Do you share a nurse-midwife's values on general health
and use of technology in childbirth?*

Chances are you will not radically change your health habits or your attitudes the moment your pregnancy is confirmed. If you are choosing a health-care provider, it is best to find someone whose outlook toward pregnancy-related issues, including the use of technology, matches yours.

Jane, for instance, loved her morning coffee. Without it, she felt like a monster. After doing some reading, she decided that going without her coffee would be worse for her pregnancy than whatever danger that amount of caffeine may have presented. Some midwives frown upon consuming any caffeine during pregnancy, and Jane did not want to feel at odds with her caregiver. But she wanted to decide these things for herself; that was foremost in her mind as she shopped for care. She found a nurse-midwife who respected her choices and helped her make informed decisions.

Equally important is that you and your caregiver share common attitudes toward technology and medical intervention in childbirth. If you are absolutely certain that you want an epidural or electronic fetal monitoring during labor, most nurse-midwife practices probably are not for you. A nurse-midwife will discuss these issues in an orientation session or by phone before you begin care.

Are you willing to accept a nurse-midwife's use of technology if she thinks it is necessary?

If you do not under any circumstances want an electronic fetal monitor, medication, or prenatal testing, a nurse-midwife may not be the right choice for you. Most will explain in advance what technology they use and under what circumstances. Do not think an exception will be made for you. If you find a nurse-midwife's approach not natural enough for your tastes, you probably should seek care elsewhere. You may be able to find another nurse-midwife or non-nurse midwife in your community whose ideas are more compatible with yours. (See

Chapters 10 and 12 for more about non-nurse mid-wives.)

Are you prepared to answer the questions and raised
eyebrows of well-meaning—and sometimes downright
nosy—friends, relatives and mere acquaintances?

Pregnant women inevitably are faced with the un-wanted pats, pokes, and advice of friends, family and strangers. If you have your baby with a nurse-midwife, especially in a community where nurse-midwives are still few in number, expect also to confront plenty of misconceptions. Laura laughs at the difference between what people expected of nurse-midwife birth and her experience in a New York hospital.

"When people asked what doctor I was going to and I said, 'I'm going to a midwife,' they looked at me in horror, as if I were going to some old witch-doctor lady and I was going to go out back and deliver over a pit!" she said.

Laura shared many of those misconceptions herself until she became pregnant and began shopping for care. After she learned that nurse-midwives are educated professionals who share her ideas about childbirth and attend births in her neighborhood hospital, she felt so good about her choice she did not mind taking the time to educate others.

Coping with grandparents-to-be may be the most difficult part for some expectant parents, especially those who are relatively young or having their first baby. What most couples find, however, is that their choice brings them new respect from friends and relatives who admire them for seeking care they believe to be right for them.

Are you comfortable with the level of monitoring?

If you feel that not using all technology available would be irresponsible, you may have qualms about rejecting continuous electronic fetal monitoring, which is not used routinely by most nurse-midwives. Experts now realize that the electronic monitors have drawbacks and may not guarantee a better outcome, but few doctors are comfortable abandoning the technology now that it is in widespread use.

*What is most important to you about your pregnancy
and birth?*

It is worth taking the time early in pregnancy—ideally, before pregnancy—to answer this question. Whether your top priority is to have a peaceful, natural experience or the most sophisticated medical technology, you are entitled to your preferences. Some women know they are at their best when they feel in control; others want to defer to authority. An issue that is a major preoccupation with the first baby—safety, often—may be supplanted by desire for a private, family-oriented birth the next time.

A WOMAN'S CHOICE

No matter how much you like the notion of nurse-midwives, no matter how much your husband or best friend believes midwife care is the way to go, if you do not feel comfortable, you are best off elsewhere. No midwife will be offended by your decision; after all, respect for a woman's choices in determining her own health care is one of nurse-midwifery's strongest credos.

If the nurse-midwife approach appeals to you, though, you owe it to yourself to find out if there exists a more satisfying way to give birth than the way your mother did, or your sister or neighbor. This search may take some effort on your part, but it is not too late even if you are a few months into your pregnancy. Most nurse-midwives will accept you well into pregnancy if you have received early care elsewhere. Early prenatal care is important, and you should not put it off because you are undecided about where or with whom to have your baby. You can switch later.

If instinct tells you that there is more to pregnancy than a growing belly, there are people who can help make the experience everything you want it to be.

"If you are looking for somebody who has the time to sit and chat, to help you deal with issues other than, Is the baby growing? Is the blood pressure normal?, then you ought to at least look at a midwife," says nurse-midwife Jan Kriebs. "And you and that midwife decide whether you fit in her practice."

FINDING A NURSE-MIDWIFE IN YOUR COMMUNITY

The most direct way to get a listing of certified nurse-midwives in your state or community is to call or write:

American College of Nurse-Midwives
1522 K Street NW, Suite 1000
Washington, D.C. 20005
202-289-0171.

Also ask for the name of the ACNM chairperson for your local area or state; she can tell you what individual practices are like.

Childbirth educators are an excellent source of information about options in your community; find them listed under "Childbirth Education" in the *Yellow Pages*. Your local chapter of LaLeche League or Healthy Mothers,

Healthy Babies, also knows about birth options where you live. Local hospitals will tell you by phone whether nurse-midwives work there. Also, look in the *Yellow Pages* under "Physicians" for Obstetricians who note they have nurse-midwives in their practices; the headings "Clinics," "Birth Centers," and "Midwives" may also have midwife listings, although they may not distinguish between certified nurse-midwives and non-nurse midwives. Some large cities, such as Los Angeles and New York, have guides to women's health and childbirth. Another good source of information is an obstetrical nurse, who will know the local scuttlebut, the reputations of doctors and midwives, and what kinds of practices they have.

Do not be afraid to look outside your general neighborhood. Once labor begins, you normally have plenty of time to get to the hospital or birth center. Even if you must drive a few minutes more to prenatal visits, you will come out ahead if you find a nurse-midwife who keeps a reliable schedule with minimal waiting room time.

The bottom line when it comes to shopping for maternity care is to ask, ask, ask. If this is your first pregnancy, you may be shy about the whole subject. Don't be. You will learn quickly that the details of childbirth are a favorite topic among the millions of women who have done it before you. Ask your friends, their friends, your colleagues, relatives, and neighbors who they went to for care, what it was like and what they thought. Then follow your instincts. Every woman is different. You are the only one who can know what is best for you.

SHOPPING FOR CARE

Whether it is for a nurse-midwife, a dentist, or a pediatrician, Denise shops. She asks friends and relatives for references, she asks people at work. And she makes an appointment, which she will pay for if charged, to talk with the caregiver.

"I know that's a scary thing for some people to do who've grown up thinking doctors have all the answers and who do not include shopping for medical care as part of the consumer movement," she said. "I don't feel that way. I know what I want out of a practitioner and I actually interview them and determine from that whether I wish to go to them."

Interviewing doctors and midwives for childbirth care is standard practice in many communities, and there is no reason to feel shy about doing it. If you have medical insurance, it probably will cover the visit. Many birth centers and hospital-based midwifery services hold free orientations.

Below are questions to ask practitioners. If you are already seeing a doctor for gynecological care, ask these questions to find out about his or her obstetrical care. If you are comparing doctors and nurse-midwives, the answers you hear may help you decide where on the spectrum of care you are most comfortable. If your care already has been chosen for you by your HMO, ask these questions anyway; the answers will give you a better idea of what to expect. Jot down questions for your visit or phone call so you will not leave anything out or get diverted in your quest for information.

Shopping for maternity care involves choosing both the place of birth and the caregiver. Some people pick the location first, then the person; others do the opposite. Usually the decision is intertwined. Chapters 8, 9, and 10 tell more about the places you can have a baby with a nurse-midwife—hospital, birth center and home—and shopping tips to help you find the one that is right for you.

QUESTIONS FOR DOCTOR OR NURSE-MIDWIFE

What is your rate of cesarean section? Episiotomy? Forceps birth? Use of drugs and anesthesia?

The answers to these questions indicate the amount of intervention during a typical childbirth. An episiotomy rate over 80 percent probably means the cut is made almost automatically, except when delivery is so rapid that there is no time. A high rate of epidural anesthesia tells you that medicated birth is the norm, perhaps even before anyone knows whether human touch and encouragement would be enough to get a woman through. And the cesarean rate indicates your likelihood of a surgical birth. Individual practices—both private practices and those in public hospitals—keep their own statistics on these elements of birth. The information provides a measure, separate from formal studies, of how those doctors and nurse-midwives work and their outcomes. As you shop, these statistics can provide you with a basis for comparing practices.

If you are interested in having your baby with the four nurse-midwives at Midwifery Services, Inc., in New York City, for instance, they can tell you that of the 146 women who began labor with them at Saint Luke's–Roosevelt Hospital in 1990, 9.6 percent had cesareans (14 women), 1.4 percent had forceps births (2 women), 60 percent gave birth with perineum intact and 40 percent had an episiotomy or tear. About 18 percent of the women requested and received epidural anesthesia, about 5 percent received analgesic pain medication and 2.7 percent received a tranquilizer. Two other women had switched to the care of a doctor prenatally.

Some doctors avoid answering these questions directly, by saying that they do the procedures only as necessary. Ask for specific numbers. Remember, you are the con-

sumer buying the doctor's services, and you have a right
to know what to expect. Do not think you will beat the
odds. If 90 percent of a doctor's patients have episiotomies, you probably will too.

Do you require or recommend prenatal testing and sonograms?

The response suggests how much input parents have
during pregnancy, and shows to what degree parents'
opinions are sought. Some women find that the doctor
who seemed relaxed about well-woman care works more
defensively when it comes to childbirth. To ensure that
they will not be blamed for a child's handicaps, some
physicians recommend testing or present it as the norm.
This attitude is something to consider if you want to make
your own testing decisions.

Who will first examine me when I get to the hospital? Who will be present during my labor?

In a standard hospital birth, your physician checks on
you briefly during labor and returns when you are ready
to push. That means your internal exam upon arrival could
be done by the hospital's on-duty nurses, interns, or
medical residents (new doctors who are in advanced
training to become obstetricians). A labor nurse is assigned to you, but hospital staffing ratios and how busy
the ward is when you begin labor dictate how much time
she actually spends by your side. If you are having your
baby with a nurse-midwife, she usually performs your
first exam; then, depending on the type of practice, she
may stay with you throughout the labor. Ask the midwife how likely it is she will have another labor at the
same time.

Find out if the doctor or nurse-midwife shares on-call

duty with someone else. If the answer is yes, do all the practitioners follow the same approach? Your doctor may be comfortable with a birthing room, but his or her partner may not be. Ask whether any promises by your doctor prior to delivery, such as no IV or no enema, will be honored by the hospital staff and other physicians.

What role will the birth partner play?

It is standard now for a father or birth partner to remain with the laboring woman throughout labor and delivery, although the amount of participation varies. Ask if he is welcome at prenatal visits and whether he can stay with the mother if he wants to in the event of a cesarean.

How much time do you allot to each prenatal visit, and how long is a typical wait in the anteroom?

A typical prenatal visit in an obstetrician's office is scheduled for no longer than fifteen minutes, although the time you spend with the doctor may be less. A nurse-midwife visit usually lasts a half hour in private practice, or slightly less in clinic settings. Look around the waiting room and ask women who are well into pregnancy how long they usually wait. If your blood pressure shoots up at every visit because the wait is making you late for work, your pregnancy, and your feelings about it, will not be enhanced.

If you feel rushed or intimidated asking these questions, do not think it will be any different a few months down the road when you want to know about protein in your diet or what you can do about your swollen ankles. On the other hand, if you find yourself getting more excited about the pregnancy as you speak with the doctor or nurse-midwife, and if he or she inspires your confidence and trust, this may be the right caregiver for you.

COMPARISON SHOPPING AMONG NURSE-MIDWIVES

By education, all nurse-midwives are created equally. But in practice, nurse-midwifery embraces a range of attitudes and approaches. The following questions will help you find the nurse-midwife that is right for you. If you already have begun care with a nurse-midwife, ask these questions anyway. The answers will give you a better picture of what lies ahead.

Whom will I see during prenatal care?

In a solo practice this is not an issue. In a medium-size practice of two, three, or four nurse-midwives, you may want to meet more than one before making your decision, because all may be involved in your care. You can often request that nearly all your prenatal care be with the same nurse-midwife.

Who will be there for the delivery?

If you feel strongly about having a nurse-midwife who knows you well at your delivery, you will be best off in a small practice. Most large practices rotate the on-call in a birth center or hospital.

What if I have a question between visits?

Find out how accessible your midwife is and the best times to call. One woman found her work schedule made it impossible for her to call during the hours designated each week for telephone questions. The problem was compounded because her nurse-midwives were trying a new schedule of fewer prenatal visits during early pregnancy. The first-time mother felt stranded without guidance for weeks at a time. This is very unusual, but worth an inquiry.

What medical conditions would require me to transfer to a doctor's care?

No woman wants to think it will happen to her, but a certain percentage of women develop the complications that require a doctor's attention. Find out in advance what your nurse-midwife's criteria are for referring a woman to a doctor's care, so you will not be surprised. If you feel strongly that you would not want to leave a midwife's care entirely, seek a practice in which midwives retain contact with a woman even after a doctor is brought in.

What is the midwife-doctor relationship?

This is one of the most important aspects of nurse-midwifery care. All nurse-midwives should have an agreement with a doctor who will care for women who develop complications, but the relationships vary. If a nurse-midwife has a written agreement with her consulting doctor, there is greater assurance that a doctor will be available in the event of a complication. Find out whether the midwife and doctor have written guidelines defining the conditions that require the doctor's involvement in pregnancy and labor.

Some nurse-midwives have a better rapport with their doctors than others. Practices in which a doctor employs the nurse-midwife, and university settings where midwives have been working for years, tend to have a high level of trust between midwives and doctors. But these nurse-midwives may have less autonomy than their self-employed colleagues. Nurse-midwives who own their practices have more independence; their relationships with doctors are more variable.

Doctors generally agree to be consultants to nurse-midwives because they consider nurse-midwifery care to be cost-efficient, safe, and satisfying for low-risk women. Doctors who work with nurse-midwives like the arrangement because they are confident that a nurse-midwife will call if there is a complication, and the women who are referred to them tend to be calm and well-informed. Doctors like having a competent caregiver available to spend time with women during routine pregnancies, leaving them free to concentrate on pathological situations. If a doctor is at all hesitant about a nurse-midwife's judgment, however, their working relationship may be strained.

Find out whether the doctor is ostracized for working with nurse-midwives. Some doctors who have worked infrequently or not at all with nurse-midwives hold common misconceptions about them, and some obstetricians have been outright hostile to nurse-midwives if they consider them a threat to their livelihoods. If doctors in your community view nurse-midwives with hostility, which is the reality in some places, you should shop more carefully for the most supportive situation available.

What will be the midwife's role if there is a problem prenatally?

Find out whether the consulting physician requires you to transfer completely to his or her practice if you develop a medical condition during pregnancy, or whether the midwife continues to be involved in your care. Will you stop seeing the nurse-midwife? Do doctor and midwife co-manage patients? Ask about financial terms: If a woman transfers to the doctor prenatally, does the doctor give credit for prenatal care already paid to the nurse-midwife? Most consulting physicians do.

What will the nurse-midwife's role be if there is a problem during labor/delivery?

Once a doctor is called in, he or she—and not the midwife—has the ultimate say on how your care will be handled. But with many physicians, the nurse-midwife remains involved. Ask whether your midwife may remain with you if you need a cesarean birth. Many doctors and hospitals allow this.

Will I meet the consulting physician? What if I don't like him or her? May I choose another physician?

Some practices and some states require at least one meeting with the physician for medical input or to acquaint you with each other if later there is an emergency during labor. Other practices leave it to the woman's choice if there is no medical reason to see the doctor. Women who did not meet the doctor until a complication arose during labor later said they wished they had taken the time to get acquainted beforehand.

What is the nurse-midwife's relationship with the hospital?

This is especially important, even if you are having your baby in a birth center or at home. All nurse-midwives who attend out-of-hospital births should either have admitting privileges at a local hospital or work with a doctor who does. If only the doctor has admitting privileges, your nurse-midwife may not be allowed to remain with you, or she may accompany you but not be involved in your care. In communities where midwives are still struggling for acceptance, there may be some hostility from the hospital's doctors and nurses. The optimum situation—and these do exist—is one in which the nurse-midwives are appreciated by the nurses and hospital staff for their competence and approach to normal birth.

Does the nurse-midwife use pain medication or anesthesia?

Some nurse-midwives introduce medication and anesthesia more readily than others. If you think you may want medication, ask about this in advance. Jane, for instance, thought she had finally found the perfect situation when she attended the hospital orientation of a nurse-midwife group that worked with a private physician: she liked the hospital, she liked the midwives and she liked their philosophy toward childbirth. Then she asked about anesthesia. She did not plan to have an epidural, but she wanted it to be available, just in case. These nurse-midwives said they did not use epidurals for vaginal birth. Jane decided to continue shopping, and eventually she found a practice that made anesthesia available.

AN INVESTMENT IN THE REST OF YOUR LIFE

Just because standard obstetrical care may have moved away from satisfying the needs of women and their families does not mean you have to resign yourself to a less than satisfying experience. It may require, though, that you apply the same amount of consumer savvy as you would for any major investment. Daniel and Jane took consumerism to its extreme when they interviewed at least six obstetricians and three nurse-midwife groups soon after Jane got pregnant. But it paid off. They found a group of nurse-midwives whose philosophy they shared and whose judgment they trusted. For something as intimate and precious as childbirth, Daniel thought that was important.

"At a certain point in every kind of expert endeavor, the data runs out, the equipment maxes out its usefulness, and sooner or later somebody has to stand at the edge of the pool, make a judgment call and jump," Daniel said. "That's the criteria we looked at: who's going to make the judgment call and do we trust the judgment?"

Pregnancy is not just a physical condition. It is an experience tied to everything else in your life, and should be viewed with no less importance. Shopping for maternity care requires a type of assertive consumerism. As two-time mother Denise found out, a safe and satisfying birth is worth the effort.

"The thing I realize is that this is a very special time for you and you are entitled to enjoy it," she said. "You are entitled to answers and you are entitled to have your fears recognized. You should go for it."

6.

A FAMILY AFFAIR

---

*"It was a lot less gory than everyone imagines it.
. . . My baby sister's eyes just lit up. It made us
feel closer to see Matthew being born—closer to
Matthew and closer to each other. You really
shouldn't have to hide these things."*
—CAROLYN, ON HER BROTHER'S BIRTH

CAROLYN WAS 13 years old when she and her sisters
Christina, 10, and Katrina, 2, watched their mother give
birth to their brother Matthew. A year and a half later
the girls still remembered with awe the magical moment
when Matthew joined the family. "We knew we were
allowed to be there," Christina said, looking back on it.
"I didn't know it was going to be that exciting."

The arrival of a new baby is significant for the whole
family. Fathers, other children, and grandparents may be
involved as much as you would like them to be, when
you have your baby with a nurse-midwife. During the
prenatal months, your nurse-midwife helps family members learn about the pregnancy and about her role in helping you. When it comes time for the birth, whether you
prefer to have an intimate experience with just your part-

ner or to surround yourself with loved ones, your nurse-midwife will help carry out your wishes.

Families that experience birth together come to regard it as the essence of their life together. Fathers feel new awe and appreciation for the female strength that brings their children into the world. Children get caught up in the excitement of welcoming "our" new baby. Grandparents love the closeness as they see their family extend into the next generation. In a time when so many forces tug families apart, family-centered birth is a celebration of family unity.

One grandfather who experienced the births of his children and grandchildren over four decades, concluded that the new trend toward family-centered birth is how childbirth ought to be. Ernest L. Boyer, president of the Carnegie Foundation for the Advancement of Teaching, described his "pilgrimage of the spirit" in a 1990 address to the American College of Nurse-Midwives, of which his wife Kay is a member.

When their first child was born, he said, he "sat forlornly in a sterile waiting room" through the wee hours of the night before he caught "a fleeting glimpse of our new baby through a hazy glass." By the time their last child was born, Kay demanded that her husband be allowed into the delivery room with her. There, Boyer said, he "began to feel the miracle and mystery of birth."

It was not until years later, when their grandchild was born at home with his own wife attending the birth, that he completed his journey. As labor progressed, the confidence and skill of his wife, another nurse-midwife, and his daughter drew his profound admiration, and he observed a spiritual strength he had never seen before. Then, as Kay placed the baby in the new mother's arms, the grandfather felt he was witnessing one of nature's greatest wonders.

"As this precious miracle of life began to nurse," he

said, "I felt the bonding and thought about how sad it is that we've removed ourselves from birth. We've turned life's most profoundly moving moments over to experts and to institutions, trusting in our inventions, rather than each other."

As families experience midwife-assisted birth they realize how natural and enriching it is for the whole family to be involved. Fathers- and grandparents-to-be who start out with doubts often turn into nurse-midwives' biggest boosters. This chapter explores your choices for involving family members in childbirth, and how families have responded to the midwife experience.

DADS

Men who start out with the notion that women have been birthing babies on their own for centuries generally are pleased from the start with the prospect of nurse-midwife care for their partners. Others may be more skeptical. "All that touchy-feely stuff is good if it makes you feel better," many fathers say, or at least think to themselves. "But shouldn't we do what is safest?"

Not all men understand the alienation some women feel with standard obstetrical and gynecological care. Not all men understand the "something's missing" feeling that comes with brisk medical checkups for a part of your body connected with emotions that are so private and complex. Learning about childbirth, learning what is normal, is the best reassurance that nurse-midwife care is safe as well as satisfying. (See Chapter 7 for studies and statistical information that prove the safety of nurse-midwifery.) Once many men become aware of exactly what the birth process entails, they find the nurse-midwife option a very sensible one. By the time the baby is born, men almost universally   describe   nurse-midwives   as   not   only   ex-

tremely skilled professionals, but also people of great em-
pathy who have a remarkable knack for making them feel
relaxed and confident.

Having your baby with a nurse-midwife means fathers
are welcome at every prenatal visit. Once labor begins,
the parents never have to be separated, and the father is
enlisted to help his partner. He may walk with her, and
provide support during a contraction. If a fetal monitor
is being used, the father can help read the strips that print
out of the machine. When the baby is finally born, the
father may be the one to lift the baby out of the birth
canal, and to cut the umbilical cord. He can hold the baby
right away. A midwife birth often ends with a peaceful
scene of mother, father, and child all dozing on the bed,
or quietly getting acquainted.

Fathers who experience birth with a nurse-midwife come
to know that this personal style of care makes having a
baby a full, safe and satisfying experience. An added bo-
nus is the feeling of closeness that gets the whole family
off to a good start together. The experiences of these fathers will give you an idea of what it is like.

Nervous Coach

In Reed's mind, a midwife was a country woman in a
long apron and cap, far removed from modern medicine.
His first visit to Childbirth Associates in Miami after his
wife Ellen became pregnant changed his mind completely. The nurse-midwife impressed him not only because she was so professional, knowledgeable, and safety
oriented, but also because of the questions *she* asked *them*.
She set out her criteria: a woman must be in excellent
health, and parents are expected to participate. That suited
Reed just fine. He liked the idea that his wife could retain
her usual good health throughout pregnancy, and he certainly wanted to be involved in the decisions. For the next
nine months, Reed went with Ellen to nearly every office

visit. He had so many questions, appointments sometimes lasted a full hour.

"Reed was scared to death of the delivery," Ellen said.
"Every time, we went over it. The midwives never got
tired of his questions and his fears."

Reed simply wanted to know the nuts and bolts of what
would happen, and he felt the nurse-midwives appreciated his interest. As a first-time father he was nervous,
and he took his coaching job very seriously.

"I wasn't sure I was going to do the right things," he
said. "I wanted to know what to expect."

The well-prepared coach came through with flying colors, as did Ellen and their 7-pound, 8-ounce daughter.
When Ellen became pregnant again, the couple actually
looked forward to sharing the experience with their midwives. Reed felt like he was returning to old friends.

"This is like a little family here, and these are the people that have hands on when we deliver," he said. "Very
personal relationships develop. These are people who really
cared about us."

Reluctant Coach

Not all expectant fathers are comfortable with the
amount of involvement expected of them. Tommy, whose
wife Laura's labor and delivery were described in Chapter
3, was 100 percent behind her choice to have a hospital
birth with a nurse-midwife. He was just not sure he could
overcome his sqeamishness about blood and hospitals.
When the midwives explained that the father could help
deliver the baby and cut the umbilical cord, he blanched.
Laura assured him that he only had to be there with her;
she did not expect him to do anything else. After all,
Tommy was the guy who fainted just from hearing a friend
describe a gashed knee over the phone.

Once labor got underway, he surprised himself. He

massaged Laura's back through each contraction. He did not balk at all once they got to the hospital. He even cut the cord.

"The whole miracle of birth, it was different than being cut open accidentally," he said. "This is a wonderful thing. We'd been going to these classes and watched a lot of videos, so I knew what it was going to look like. It was the most natural kind of thing. We couldn't have asked for anything better. It was almost unreal."

Getting Closer

Although no man can feel those contractions, being close to his partner throughout childbirth strengthens a couple's bond as they embark on parenthood together. In a time when men and families are redefining fatherhood to include more interaction between father and child, a father's involvement at birth is a chance to be a part of the baby's life from the start.

For Donald, assisting at the birth of his second daughter, described in Chapter 1, was a "fun experience, very gratifying" and a time to be close to his wife. Although the birth was in a hospital, there were no tubes and electronic devices between him and Nancy as she reached the final stages of labor. He described it as "a tremendous interaction with your spouse," made easier by the nurse-midwife. She was there for technical expertise, making sure all was well and paving the way for his involvement.

As the baby's head crowned, Donald moved from the head of the bed for the first glimpse of his child. After the midwife eased out the head and shoulders, Donald took over, tucking his hands under his daughters tiny arms to lift her out of the birth canal and onto Nancy's belly. For Donald, that was a moment of sheer, exhilarating pleasure. And the midwife made it "so darn comfortable."

"It's not just *someone* who is with you. It's your birthing person," he said. "You actually develop a tremendous rapport."

Like many fathers, Donald recommends being as involved in the birth as possible, for the simple satisfaction and pleasure it brings and for the way the experience strengthens a man's bond to his family.

"There's no reason why delivery shouldn't be part of the experience of having a child," Donald said. "Being a father is not just going to ballets and outings."

A Calming Influence

During labor, the constant presence of the nurse-midwife takes pressure off a nervous father. Most men, no matter how well prepared, have fear about the birth itself. Knowing that the nurse-midwife will detect any problems, a father can concentrate on soothing his partner.

"If your wife says rub my feet, you rub her feet; if she says leave the room, you leave the room," said Craig, a veteran of three births at a birth-center and one at home. "She's the one who has to go through it. You make her birth experience as pleasant as possible."

As the force of childbirth takes over a woman's body, the last person she may want to see is the fellow who helped get her into this situation. One mother firmly told her partner, a diligent breathing coach, to take his "who-who-whos" and "hee-hee-hees" somewhere else.

"During transition, the woman will blame everything on you—world hunger and all. She'll be screaming and cursing," Craig said.

That is when a nurse-midwife is especially helpful. It is comforting for a man to know that the person attending his wife is someone they both trust, to comfort her as well as detect problems. At that moment a midwife is part of your family. Over and over again, fathers marvel at how their midwife balanced skilled professionalism with nurturing, to help the whole family.

A FATHER'S VIEW, AWE AND ENVY

Ted had already seen the high-tech birth of his first child, with impersonal staff in a hospital room that he found sterile and alienating. At the birth of his second child, however, with nurse-midwives in a birth center, he saw a whole different view of birth:

> When my wife's contractions were at their worst, when she was having trouble keeping her concentration on the breathing and away from the pain, occurred a moment that crystallized the experience at the birthing center. Connie was in a chair and I was perched next to her holding her hand. Kneeling in front of Connie were the nurse-midwife and nurse. The nurse held Connie's other hand, the midwife stroked her hair, and they both were leaning close, gently telling her they were with her, to hang on, they were going to get her through this contraction, the one after, and the one after that.
>
> And Connie heard them, and she believed them, and she drew strength from them. It was a sisterhood so tight that I had no hope, or desire, of penetrating. I sat there holding her hand feeling very invisible and useless and watched in awe and envy. Men would never, could never, get this close. I felt like I had been allowed a look into the spirit of motherhood. The moment passed, but I will always remember it.

SIBLINGS

In some hospitals, and in nearly all birth centers and home births, chilldren are permitted to attend the birth if parents wish. How to prepare children for a birth in the family and whether to include them in the birth itself are difficult questions for many parents. To prepare your child, your nurse-midwife will suggest or lend books and videos that explain birth to youngsters. She may refer you to a sibling preparation class at a hospital or birth center.

When it comes to deciding whether to have children at the birth, some women are concerned that a young child would be traumatized by seeing and hearing his or her mother in the throes of labor, and that an older child would be embarrassed. Some are concerned about exposing youngsters to the blood of childbirth. You know yourself and your child best. If you think your child's presence will make it difficult for you to concentrate on the labor, or if you think your distress may alarm him or her, arrange in advance for the child to be elsewhere. You can plan to have the whole family together soon after the birth.

If you think you might like to have your children with you though, your nurse-midwife will encourage you. Children who are prepared take birth very much in stride, regardless of their age or gender. Some remain nonchalant once the great event begins, preferring a good cartoon in the next room to the actual birth. Other children are simply enchanted.

If you plan to have your children with you, your nurse-midwife will require that they be accompanied by a grandparent, babysitter or other familiar adult. That rule holds firm, even if you have only one other child, and even if the birth is in your own home. Birth requires all the attention of the woman in labor, her partner and the nurse-midwife. An extra person is crucial to keep children busy, to answer questions and to prepare meals and snacks.

If you plan to have your child with you, do not be surprised if he or she is not much interested. Labor is long and boring for children. Make sure they are free to come and go; children should not be expected to remain in the labor room if they seem uneasy or bored there. They should also be comfortable with your nurse-midwife. Bring school-age children by the office to meet the nurse-midwife toward the end of pregnancy. Younger children who attend prenatal visits become comfortable with the midwife and learn about pregnancy along the way. By the time of the birth, they have heard the baby's heartbeat and are prepared for what will happen.

A nurse-midwife is an expert at setting the tone for a calm, family-centered birth. Once labor is underway, she may chat with the children during the pauses between contractions. "Isn't Mommy making funny noises, she's really working hard," is how one nurse-midwife explains the grunts and groans of labor. Small children pick up on the cues of people around them. If the atmosphere is loving and happy, children usually are too, adding their own unpredictable exuberance.

"OKAY EVERYBODY—BREATHE!"

"I'll never forget the looks on each of my little girls' faces," said Doris, describing what she saw when she raised her eyes after that final push. Carolyn, Christina, and Katrina were spellbound at Matthew's arrival.

Doris wanted the whole family together for the birth, her first with nurse-midwives in a birth center. To prepare the girls, she explained straightforwardly to all of them, even two-year-old Katrina, the mechanics of labor and birth, and what probably would happen once they got to the birth center.

"As open and honest and natural as a mother tells her kids, that is how they take it," she said. "It prevents a lot of discomfort or uneasiness."

When Doris's contractions began on a weekday morning, a friend picked up the older girls at school. Doris's husband met them en route, and the whole family piled into one car for the ride to the birth center. On the way, contractions became a family affair.

"I'd say, 'Okay everybody—breathe!' Doris said. "And we were all laughing."

During five hours of labor at the birth center, the girls played together in the family room, occasionally joining their parents in the birth room next door. It was a relaxed time with the whole family together, and everyone could take part. When the midwife rubbed Doris's back, Katrina joined in, toddling up from behind to give a backrub to the midwife. When the baby crowned, all three sisters gathered around to watch.

"Weird and nice," was how Christina, 10, described the birth. Carolyn, 13, was surprised at how little blood there was. She especially loved watching Katrina's amazement as their brother was being born, and how being together at such an important time drew the whole family closer.

For her older daughters, Doris thought the experience added a realistic dimension to what most adolescents learn about sexuality. She did not anticipate the unity it would foster among her children.

"They feel a sense of responsibility for each other," she said. "There's nothing they wouldn't do for each other. Being together as a family during the birth experience nurtured that. It isn't just like Mommy and Daddy are doing this, and bringing you a brother or sister."

"HERE'S MY BABY!"

All sixteen couples whose children were present at the birth of a sibling in a New England community hospital said they would have their children with them again if they had a subsequent birth, a 1985 study in the *Journal of Nurse-Midwifery* reported. Many said the older children made the experience more joyful, and added a feeling of family completeness. One mother could never have anticipated the war whoop of YEA! that rose in the room as soon as the baby was born. Her five-year-old son burst into a spontaneous chorus of "Happy Birthday," and everyone else joined in.[1]

Children often immediately cleave to the newborn, climbing right onto the bed with their mother to hold or touch their little brother or sister. The presence of children at a birth may diminish sibling rivalry, because the older brother or sister never feels left out. In a study of twenty-two families, published in 1986 in *Birth*, mothers reported that children who attended the birth of a sibling showed more positive behaviors toward the new baby than children who were not at the birth.[2]

Nurse-midwife Leslie Stewart, who works in a home birth practice in Los Angeles, tells of the four-year-old who could hardly wait for the new baby to arrive. Her mother, at the end of a long labor, was using the hands-and-knees position to relieve pressure on her tailbone. In that position, the baby's head was born. One more push and the body would be out. As dad and midwife concentrated on coaching the mother, little Ellie slipped by. Before anyone could catch her, she planted a kiss smack on the forehead of her half-born brother. "Here's my baby!" she announced. That was one child born into a room full of family love and laughter.

GRANDPARENTS

Not everyone is comfortable at first with the notion of nurse-midwives or family-centered birth, especially after two or three generations during which birth was "women's business" in the hands of doctors—removed from sight and not much talked about. Almost inevitably, grandparents-to-be will have an avalanche of questions and concerns about nurse-midwife care. Some expectant grandmothers are perplexed by this "new" way of care, having been told thirty years earlier that heavy medication and medical intervention were the safest and most modern options. If your parents or in-laws are interested enough, help them learn and feel comfortable about your choice. Let them see just what a nurse-midwife does. Suggest that your mother or mother-in-law join you for a prenatal visit or a tour of the maternity ward or birth center. Lend her this book.

Nurse-midwives are accustomed to grandmothers-to-be who sit quietly through most of a prenatal visit, then overflow with questions. That's fine with them—ask away. A nurse-midwife wants the whole family to have confidence in her care.

"It's my challenge, by the end of the visit, to have her completely comfortable and satisfied about what is happening with her daughter," nurse-midwife Barbara Brennan says.

Some people are reluctant to tell their parents at all that they are having their baby with a nurse-midwife, especially if they feel that their parents tend to be critical of decisions they make. Often, though, the choice of a nurse-midwife sparks surprising revelations from their own mothers about their frustrations when they gave birth years earlier—the haze of drugs, the loss of control, and the separation from their families and their babies. Many grandparents-to-be who do not start out supportive of the nurse-midwife option come to respect their children for following their own convictions about what is best for them and their baby.

One new grandmother advises others to find out about nurse-midwives before voicing any objections. She herself had some reservations when she heard that her son and daughter-in-law planned to have their baby with a nurse-midwife. Without telling them, she went on her own to see the birthing suites in the hospital where they planned to have the baby. She wanted to get a better idea of what nurse-midwife birth would be like.

"If you can't be completely supportive, don't damage it, don't influence it," she said. "Learn about it."

Satisfied about safety issues, the grandmother was proud that her daughter-in-law "had the courage to be an innovator." When her own children were born some thirty years earlier, she had been concerned about the effects of medication on them and on her, but she felt she had little choice. She was secretly glad that during three of the five births the medication did not take, leaving her wide awake. But her husband was not allowed in the delivery room with her. She liked knowing it could be different for her son and daughter-in-law.

"Seeing this happen now makes me feel that new does not always mean better," she said. "This is better. What makes it better is that a woman has another option."

A generation ago, some women received very little information about what actually went on during birth. Many gave birth to a family full of children without learning much about the process. That was the case with Louise's mother. When Louise told her that she would be having her first baby in a Denver birth center, she reacted cautiously. So Louise invited her to a childbirth class at the center to see what it was all about. As the class ended, her mother wanted to know much more.

"She asked a million questions," Louise said. "She had six kids and never saw any of them being born."

Louise's mother attended the birth—in many ways the

first she was truly a part of. She beamed as she watched the birth of her grandson.

"She's close like this with my son," Louise said, crossing her index and middle fingers. "And I'm sure it's because she saw him being born."

Even though nurse-midwives allow grandparents to attend the birth, the decision whether to have them there is strictly yours. No matter how much your mother or mother-in-law hints, or your cousin, sister, or best friend, for that matter, if you do not think you will be comfortable with that person at the labor and delivery, politely say so. Birth is something you can share with family and friends, but ultimately the birth is yours. It is up to you to decide who you want with you.

7.

A STRONG RECORD OF HEALTHY BABIES

"The weight of evidence indicates that, within their areas of competence . . . Certified Nurse-Midwives provide care whose quality is equivalent to that of care provided by physicians. Moreover, . . . CNMs are more adept than physicians at providing services that depend on communication with patients and preventive actions."
—U. S. CONGRESS, OFFICE OF TECHNOLOGY ASSESSMENT, 1986.[1]

YOU LIKE THE NOTION of low-intervention birth in theory. You feel a nurse-midwife's personal attention and demeanor will keep you calm emotionally. But when it comes to a rational look at safety, both yours and your baby's, is a nurse-midwife really the right way to go? Study after study conclude that the answer is yes.

Nurse-midwives were introduced in the United States to improve maternal and infant health in places where there were not enough doctors and nurses. The first studies of nurse-midwifery here showed that, indeed, prematurity, infant deaths, and maternal deaths all decreased when nurse-midwives were introduced. In subsequent years, as nurse-midwifery care became the choice of more and more informed women, researchers began comparing this care with top drawer obstetrical care. This chapter cites studies done by nurse-midwives, obstetricians, and public health experts which show that nurse-midwife care leads to equally good outcomes with less intervention.

Now that the benefits of nurse-midwifery are clear, researchers are focusing on the components of that care, looking at which elements are most effective and why. The body of research continues to build, showing not only that nurse-midwives present a safe alternative for healthy women, but also that they hold distinct advantages over standard obstetrical care. Those women with risk factors from family, social, or economic situations benefit additionally from the extra attention and love provided by certified nurse-midwives.

QUALITY CONTROL

Nurse-midwives monitor their own profession closely. The American College of Nurse-Midwives (ACNM) expects all members to participate in regularly scheduled peer review, a process in which nurse-midwives review each other's practices and outcomes. A panel of nurse-midwives looks at the charts describing care given to individual women, and questions whether problems were identified promptly and handled correctly, and whether the results were good for mother and child. Most nurse-midwives eagerly participate either through a review arranged by their local ACNM chapter or through an informal arrangement with other nurse-midwives. Peer review is not required by law; it is something nurse-midwives have instituted for themselves. Many nurse-mid-wives also keep their own statistics of births, which provide a base for comparison outside of formal studies.

The American College of Nurse-Midwives also maintains a strict disciplinary procedure for anyone practicing outside the norm. If any patient, doctor, or other nurse-midwife feels that a nurse-midwife is practicing unsafely or in violation of professional ethics, he or she can file a grievance with ACNM. That sets in motion a disciplinary investigation that can result in a nurse-midwife losing her certification. Nurse-midwives as a profession believe it is important to maintain strict standards of care. Grievances are taken seriously.

A HISTORY OF HEALTHIER MOTHERS, HEALTHIER BABIES

One of the first published reports of midwifery care in the United States looked at 4,988 home births to low-income women cared for by nurse-midwives of the Maternity Center Association in New York City from 1931 to 1951. The report of the Maternity Center, published in the *American Journal of Obstetrics and Gynecology* in 1955, showed that 98 percent of the women delivered their babies safely at home, including 86 breech babies and 5 multiple births.[2]

At the Frontier Nursing Service in Kentucky from 1925 to 1954, neonatal and maternal death rates and prematurity rates were considerably lower than national averages, despite the fact that most of the births were at home in conditions of extreme poverty.[3]

One of the landmark studies of nurse-midwifery care showed that the health of mothers and babies improved when nurse-midwives began working at Madera County Hospital in rural California. In response to a shortage of health-care workers, two nurse-midwives were hired in July 1960 to provide prenatal care and assist women in labor. Physicians were available for complications. Three years later, an assessment of the program showed prematurity and infant death had dropped, more mothers were coming for prenatal care, and more were returning for the routine exam six weeks after birth. At the end of three years, however, the state's doctors refused to back a state law that would have allowed nurse-midwives to practice as they had in the pilot program. The gains made during the pilot program promptly deteriorated. During the three years after the program ended, neonatal death rose from 10.3 per 1,000 births during the program to 32.1 per 1,000 births. Prenatal care decreased and premature births rose. Writing in the *American Journal of Obstetrics and Gynecology* in 1976, researchers concluded that the "lower quantity and probably lower quality of care" after the nurse-midwives departed were the main causes of the subsequent increased prematurity and infant death.[4]

COMPARING DOCTOR AND NURSE-MIDWIFE CARE

These studies all suggested that bringing nurse-midwives to places where care was inadequate brought good results for mothers and babies. The next step was to evaluate nurse-midwife care as an alternative to standard obstetrical care. This began during the 1970s, as affluent women began seeking out nurse-midwives, and health administrators realized that nurse-midwives were cost-effective. Researchers began comparing the outcomes of nurse-midwife births to physician care in the same populations.

At the University of Mississippi Medical Center in 1972 and 1973, 438 low-risk women were randomly assigned

either to a team of nurse-midwives (with physician consultation) or the usual hospital team of obstetricians and
residents. The two groups showed equal outcomes
throughout their care, with two exceptions. Women assigned to nurse-midwives attended more prenatal visits—
94 percent of appointments were kept, compared to 80
percent with physicians—and women with nurse-midwives had fewer forceps deliveries. The researchers concluded that nurse-midwives should be allowed to care for
low-risk women, thereby meeting the demand for family-centered care and leaving doctors free to concentrate
on women at higher medical risk.[5]

In another hospital, 85 low-risk women admitted in labor were randomly assigned either to nurse-midwives or
to the more traditional physician team. Nurse-midwives
showed less routine use of electronic fetal monitoring and
intravenous fluids, smaller doses of anesthesia and pain
medication, and fewer episiotomies. Women in the midwife group also had a shorter second stage of labor. Length
of hospital stay and infant Apgar scores, which gauge infant health one minute and five minutes after birth, were
the same.[6]

THE PHILADELPHIA STORY

One of the most thorough comparisons of nurse-midwife
care versus standard obstetrical care was done by analyzing 1,600 births at two Philadelphia hospitals. At the
family-oriented Booth Maternity Center, certified nurse-
midwives (with physician consultation) provided prenatal, labor and delivery assistance, and newborn care.
Thomas Jefferson University Hospital is a top-level specialty hospital—called a tertiary hospital—where medical

KAISER PERMANENTE—NURSE-MIDWIVES
AN "UNQUALIFIED SUCCESS" IN
SOUTHERN CALIFORNIA HMO

When Kaiser Permanente Medical Center in Anaheim, California, formed its obstetrics and gynecology department in 1980, it devised a team approach using doctors, nurse-practitioners, and nurse-midwives for the affluent, suburban clientele of their health maintenance organization. Nurse-midwives and nurse-practitioners handled nearly all of the care, including deliveries, for normal pregnancies—about 57 percent of all maternity patients. Obstetricians devoted most of their time to women with complications.

Three years into the program, its leaders compared results with other nearby hospitals that did not use nurse-midwives. Health outcomes for mothers and babies were the same. And the care was cost efficient: hospital costs were between $34 and $223 less per birth when compared to seven other Kaiser hospitals.

A phone survey showed that few women considered themselves knowledgeable about nurse-midwives before receiving care. Afterward nearly all felt confident in a nurse-midwife's ability to deliver a baby. On a scale of one to five, 93 percent of patients rated their satisfaction with nurse-midwives as a four or five.

Organizers of the program reported these findings in the *American Journal of Obstetrics and Gynecology,* and concluded that using nurse-midwives as part of an obstetrical team was "an unqualified success."

"Once certified nurse-midwives are introduced to patients," the authors wrote, "it is clear that including certified nurse-midwives on the obstetric team is one of the rare ways in which a cheaper model of health-care delivery becomes the option most preferred by nearly all concerned."[7]

school graduates complete their training. A random sample of 796 women who gave birth at Booth in 1977 and 1978 were matched with 804 women at Jefferson who gave birth at the same time for age, race, obstetrical history, and education.

One of the most significant differences was a higher cesarean section rate at Thomas Jefferson—18.2 percent compared to 5.3 percent at Booth.[8] Noting that use of forceps and cesareans were associated with heavy babies at Jefferson but not at Booth, researchers speculated that at the maternity hospital a large fetus was not commonly considered reason for these procedures.[9] Delivery by outlet forceps, the type used when the baby is low in the vaginal opening, was three times greater at Jefferson.[10] Fetal distress and maternal age over thirty, questionable reasons for surgical birth, were more likely to be the reason for a cesarean at Jefferson. For a condition such as maternal bleeding, which more clearly calls for a cesarean, rates were the same.[11]

Illness among newborns and the percentage of women with fever during labor and immediately after were lower at Booth, and babies born there weighed more. Women and infants had shorter hospital stays in Booth. A higher percentage of infants born at Booth, however, needed resuscitation or scored lower than the good-health threshold of 7 on the one-minute Apgar test; the researchers concluded this was due to the greater reluctance of the nurse-midwife than the physician to intervene in a labor and delivery that was progressing normally. But by the five-minute Apgar test, scores at the two hospitals were similar, leaving researchers to further conclude that whatever disadvantage resulted from less intervention in labor and delivery disappeared within minutes. There were no differences in newborn mortality rates.

Writing in the journal *Medical Care* in 1988, researchers concluded: "The assumption that maternity care provided in the tertiary hospital is the 'best' must be reevaluated in other studies of low-risk pregnant women. It may represent only one model of 'quality care.' " Their second conclusion was that "we cannot presume that use of obstetric procedures necessarily decrease the risk of poor outcomes."[12]

A separate evaluation of the same births showed that obstetric procedures were used more frequently at Jefferson. Episiotomies were done on 64.8 percent of Jefferson women, compared to 43 percent at Booth. At Booth, 21.1 percent had a tear but no cut; at Jefferson the rate was 5.5 percent. Generally, the tears at Jefferson were more severe. Pain medication, without anesthesia, was used more often at Booth; anesthesia, without pain medication, was used more often at Jefferson. The hospitals had similar rates of inducing labor.[13]

The most marked difference in number of procedures done showed up among low-risk women, pointing out perhaps the most significant difference between the approaches of the two hospitals. For high-risk women, the two hospitals had similar rates for most obstetric procedures, although invasive delivery and anesthesia were slightly more likely at Jefferson. Low-risk women, however, were far more likely to receive anesthesia or invasive delivery at Jefferson. These women were four times more likely to have a prenatal x-ray, labor stimulation, or electronic monitoring at Jefferson; they were 12 times more likely to have forceps or cesarean and 22 times more likely to have anesthesia than low-risk women at Booth.[14]

The researchers concluded in a 1984 study in *Obstetrics and Gynecology* that Jefferson's role as a teaching hospital may have contributed to the higher rate of intervention there. At Booth, intervention was kept at a minimum for low-risk women, the researchers noted, but in a teaching hospital like Jefferson, even when intervention was not required for medical reasons, "The use of procedures that carry little risk to the woman or the fetus may be considered appropriate and desirable for teaching purposes." [15]

GOOD SENSE MAKES GOOD SCIENCE

No one really knows the ideal combination of testing, monitoring and intervention for pregnancy and labor. But clear evidence that nurse-midwife care produces good results, cost savings and high satisfaction for women has prompted researchers to look more carefully at what causes nurse-midwifery to work so well.

Much of what nurse-midwives do is based on good sense, instinct, and a long history of learning what works best. Now research is validating the effectiveness of some of these practices. Taking castor oil to stimulate labor, for instance, is an age-old practice that many nurse-midwives suggest to encourage an overdue labor, but some people doubted its effectiveness. In 1984, a study published in the *Journal of Nurse-Midwifery* compared the experiences of 196 women whose water broke before contractions began. Of the 107 women who then took castor oil, 75 percent went into labor spontaneously within 24 hours—compared to 58 percent of those who did not take castor oil. Those who did not begin labor within 24 hours were induced with synthetic oxytocin. The nurse-midwife who conducted the study concluded that castor oil is a safe and effective way to stimulate labor. [16]

The hands-on approach of nurse-midwives has also been assessed in a study. Thirty women, interviewed soon after normal vaginal birth with a nurse-midwife, said that touch helped them cope with labor. Simple hand-holding was valued most, because it conveyed feelings of sympathy, participation, encouragement, and even pain relief. [17]

Other studies have looked at the value of allowing parents to be with the baby right after birth. Researchers found that allowing a father to have physical contact with the baby immediately after birth expedited the acquaintance process and enhanced bonds of affection with the newborn.[18] Another study of 187 first-time, low-income mothers was done to gauge whether rooming-in—the practice of allowing the baby to remain in the mother's hospital room, rather than in the nursery—helped them become more attached to their babies. Of the women, 72 delivered before the hospital allowed rooming-in, 80 received rooming-in, and 35 requested but did not receive rooming-in. All the babies were healthy, all the births were normal. Based on observations during an infant feeding, rooming-in mothers showed more signs of attachment to their newborns than the two other groups.[19]

A CLOSER LOOK

Recent research has also focused on the effectiveness of the routine interventions that nurse-midwives try to avoid. A 1985 review in the *Journal of Nurse-Midwifery* of all studies on postdate pregnancies, for instance, found no evidence that outcomes for mother or baby were better when labor was automatically *induced* because the fetus had reached a predetermined gestational age.[20]

In 1985, a study published in the journal *Birth* compared women who received *epidural anesthesia* with those who used other pain relief or no medication at all. The study found that women who received epidural anesthesia had longer labors, needed Pitocin more frequently to augment labor, had a higher incidence of forceps deliveries and more bladder catheterizations.[21] Two years later a study in the same journal found that among 70 women questioned, only 27 percent said the experience of labor matched their expectations. Their most frequent surprise: gettting less pain relief than expected from medication.[22]

During the 1980s numerous studies looked into whether continuous *electronic fetal monitoring* truly had the expected benefits over checks of the baby's heartbeat with a fetoscope at regular intervals. The author of a 1990 editorial in the *New England Journal of Medicine* summarized studies of continuous electronic fetal monitoring and concluded the answer was no.

"Clearly the hoped-for benefit from intrapartum electronic fetal monitoring has not been realized," Dr. Roger Freeman of Memorial Medical Center in Long Beach, California, wrote. "It is unfortunate that randomized, controlled trials were not carried out before this form of technology became universally applied. . . . The story of electronic fetal monitoring also illustrates the need for proper randomized clinical trials before new forms of technology are introduced that may become the standard practice without clearly demonstrated benefit."[23]

Traditional reasons for doing an *episiotomy* have been to avoid a dangerous tear for the mother and to limit trauma for the infant. A 1981 study in the *Journal of Nurse-Midwifery,* however, showed that five-minute Apgar scores were not notably different when the head was delivered slowly over an intact perineum, and one-minute scores were actually higher.[24] In the same journal, a 1985 report on 100 normal births in which no episiotomy was made showed that 67 women had no lacerations at all, 16 had abrasions that needed no repair, and 17 required stitches. None had serious tears. All babies had Apgar scores of 9 or 10 at five minutes after birth.[25] A 1991 study of 367 women who had normal, vaginal deliveries showed that women who had episiotomies had a higher rate of delayed perineal healing (7.7 percent) due to separation of the wound or infection than the no-episiotomy group (2.2 percent); slow healing was also more common in women who had episiotomies than those who experienced lacerations.[26]

An analysis of *vaginal birth after cesarean* (VBAC) at Booth Maternity Center from 1976 to 1981, published in *Birth,* showed that 78.6 percent of women who attempted labor after a prior cesarean were successful at vaginal birth.[27] A study of a Minnesota nurse-midwifery service, published in the *Journal of Nurse-Midwifery* in 1989 showed that 83 percent of all women attempting VBAC at an in-hospital birth center were successful. The authors concluded that nurse-midwives could safely manage vaginal birth after cesarean, with appropriate physician consultation and available hospital services.[28]

THE NATIONAL BIRTH CENTER STUDY

One of the strongest endorsements of nurse-midwifery care came in 1989, when the prestigious *New England Journal of Medicine* published the results of a massive study of 11,814 births that began at 84 of the nation's birth centers, most of them operated by nurse-midwives. The size of the study and its sound research techniques provided a window into the efficacy of nurse-midwifery, with a low (4 percent) rate of cesarean section, good outcomes and high maternal satisfaction.[29] More details of the study are explained in Chapter 9.

GOVERNMENT CALLS FOR MORE USE OF NURSE-MIDWIVES

By the late 1980s concern about inadequate prenatal care in the U.S. produced a flurry of government reports, nearly all of which suggested increasing the use of nurse-mid-

REACHING TEENS

Nurse-midwives have clearly distinguished themselves as being able to improve the outcomes of teen pregnancies. Teenagers are more vigilant about keeping their prenatal appointments when they are seeing a nurse-midwife; and every visit is an opportunity for the midwife to encourage good eating habits and warn against the cigarettes, alcohol, and drugs that inhibit healthy fetal growth. This is crucial because low birthweight, one of the biggest problems for babies born to teens, can result in expensive and damaging health problems.

A study of pregnant teens in South Carolina published in 1985 in the *Journal of Nurse-Midwifery* showed that those whose care included a nurse-midwife had a low birthweight rate of 9 percent, compared to 13 percent of teens matched by age, race, socioeconomic status, and medical risk statewide.[30]

The same year, the *Journal* also reported results from a Chicago nurse-midwifery service for adolescents. Outcomes for 947 pregnant teens there included a lower rate of underweight babies than among similar teens in the city, state and nationwide. Worth noting is that the cesarean rate was only 6.8 percent.[31]

wives as a way to reach more women and reduce the rate of low-birthweight babies. The National Academy of Science's Institute of Medicine in its 1985 report *Preventing Low Birthweight* called for more reliance on nurse-midwives. The authors noted that nurse-midwives were particularly effective in caring for pregnant women at high risk of low birthweight for social and economic reasons because they "tend to relate to their patients in a nonauthoritarian manner and to emphasize education, support and patient satisfaction." Women cared for by nurse-midwives tend to keep their appointments more regularly and follow the advice given. The authors concluded, "Maternity programs designed to serve high-risk mothers should increase their use of these providers; and state laws should be supportive of nurse-midwife practice."[32]

The following year, the U.S. Congress Office of Technology Assessment reported to the Senate Committee on Appropriations that nurse-midwives could provide care equal to that of physicians for low-risk women, and noted the superior communication between nurse-midwives and their patients. The report acknowledged the evidence that nurse-midwives have provided effective and low-cost care in underserved areas, and recommended using CNMs rather than physicians as a cost-effective way to extend maternity care.[33]

In 1988, an Institute of Medicine committee described the maternity care system in the U.S. as "fundamentally flawed, fragmented and overly complex" in the report *Prenatal Care: Reaching Mothers, Reaching Infants*. The authors called for a new system that relied on both physicians and nurse-midwives, citing the proven effectiveness of nurse-midwives with low-income women, the lower cost of nurse-midwives compared to physicians, and the shortage of physicians willing to work in public clinics. They also pointed out that some Hispanic and Asian women find it unacceptable to have a pelvic exam done by a man. The committee recommended: increased use of certified nurse-midwives and obstetrical nurse-practitioners, government and physician support for collaboration between physicians and nurse-midwives, and uniform laws governing nurse-midwives in all states.[34]

The same year, the National Commission to Prevent Infant Mortality urged a plan of action to improve access to prenatal care, including more doctors and certified nurse-midwives in underserved communities and recommended expanding nurse-midwifery education in state universities.[35]

As nurse-midwives are being sought by women and families across the economic spectrum, the government has realized that the care they offer is a cost-effective, high-quality way to give a healthy start to all babies.

8.

HOSPITAL BIRTH
WITH A NURSE-MIDWIFE

"With a nurse-midwife in a hospital, I was just completely covered. I could have everything I wanted. I could have all the high-tech nonsense that I might need, but still have that security, that wonderful, supportive feeling you get from the nurse-midwives. I could have it all."

—KAREN, A MOTHER

"THE BEST OF both worlds" is how Karen and other mothers describe having a baby with a nurse-midwife in a hospital. Plenty of doctors and nurse-midwives agree. Many women know at the outset that they want a nurse-midwife birth, but they are not comfortable with the prospect of having a baby outside a hospital. Although the vast majority of births are uncomplicated and do not need the medical assistance that a hospital offers, many parents feel better just knowing it is there. More than 80 percent of births attended by nurse-midwives take place in hospitals. In a large, busy hospital, if a complication develops that requires a cesarean, you can be in the operating room in less time than it takes for the doctor to scrub up. (Community hospitals may take somewhat longer to assemble the anesthesiologist, the technicians, etc.). Hospitals that specialize in obstetrics have newborn intensive care units and specialists available around the clock.

You have already read about what a nurse-midwife does during labor and delivery; this chapter explains how her actions and approach fit into a hospital setting. It tells you what to expect during a nurse-midwife birth in a hospital and how the experience may differ from hospital birth with a doctor. Finally, it offers tips to help you shop for a hospital.

NO "BIRTH PLAN" NECESSARY

In the 1970s, as families began asserting their ideas of how they wanted birth to be, a common strategy was to draw up a birth plan. The birth plan detailed a family's preferences for the birth, with a list of dos and don'ts for the hospital staff, to avoid unnecessary medical intrusion. Some people made very specific instructions: what pain relief could be used and under what circumstances; to be given liquids instead of an IV; not to give a bottle of sugar water to the baby in the nursery when the mother plans to breastfeed. Parents felt that this piece of paper, signed and left with the hospital staff, gave the family control in defining the birth they wanted—the basic premise being that the hospital's usual policies were contrary to the family's wishes.

When you have a baby with a nurse-midwife in a hospital, there is no need for this type of written birth plan. You have discussed your preferences with your nurse-midwife. She knows your thoughts on pain medication, and you know she will not use certain interventions unless absolutely necessary. There won't be any surprises, even if the nurse-midwife you saw most often in prenatal care is not the one with you for the delivery. You know what to expect because nurse-midwives in the same practice share the same approach. Any requests you make in advance will be noted on your chart and honored by whomever is with you for the birth.

In some hospitals, women giving birth with a nurse-midwife follow different procedures from other women by an agreement worked out between the nurse-midwife and the hospital. For instance, in a hospital that requires all laboring women to have an IV and continuous electronic fetal monitoring, a nurse-midwife may arrange for these interventions to be left to her discretion. Many hospitals allow such deviations from their rules because of nurse-midwives' good track record for keeping exceptionally close watch on their patients and seeking help if complications develop.

ARRIVING AT THE HOSPITAL

Your nurse-midwife will probably have you preregister with the hospital, so that when you arrive in labor, you bypass most paperwork and waiting. In a typical situation, your nurse-midwife has told the hospital that you are on your way, and you are directed straight to your room. Chances are, your nurse-midwife will arrive before you do. She will help you into a hospital gown or whatever you brought to wear and take your vital signs: blood pressure, pulse, baby's heart rate. She will perform a vaginal exam to tell her—and you—how many centimeters your cervix has dilated.

Health maintenance organizations and public health programs have nurse-midwives in the hospital around the clock, generally on twelve-hour shifts. If you are in one of these programs, you deliver with whichever nurse-midwife is on duty when you arrive; it will probably be someone you saw at least once for a prenatal visit. If your nurse-midwife is in private practice, she or the midwife on-call meets you at the hospital after you have decided, by phone, that you are in active labor. In either case, a nurse-midwife will plan to remain with you from the time you arrive until after your baby is born.

When you arrive at the hospital, if it seems that you are still in early labor, your nurse-midwife may perform the internal exam before formally admitting you. If you are dilated only two or three centimeters, she may not admit you yet. She may send you home or point you to a nearby park or shopping mall with marching orders—literally. No matter how excited you are for your baby finally to be born, if the event is obviously many hours away, there is no need for you to become bored and anxious while walking the hospital halls. If all is well, you are better off doing your walking through a more scenic and relaxing route.

What happens once you are admitted depends on how close you are to having your baby and how uncomfortable you are. If you are far from the pushing stage, you may be urged to get up off the bed and move around, since the activity spurs labor. You may unpack your personal things, arrange the extra pillows you brought and turn on the music you planned for your labor. You may walk the halls with your partner or nurse-midwife. These activities may not be the norm in other hospital rooms, for other women, but when a nurse-midwife is handling the birth, labor proceeds in this relaxed, personal way with the natural rhythms of your own labor setting the pace. As long as everything is going normally, *you* decide whether you prefer to be walking, in the shower, or rocking in a chair. *You* create an environment for your own comfort. Just because birth is taking place in a large institution, it need not be impersonal.

A SINGLE FLOW

As hospital care evolved through the middle of this century, it came to mean a marathon of room changes for the mother. Women were instructed to come to the hospital when contractions started. They were examined in a triage or admitting room and then spent hours in a labor room—medicated, in bed, and checked periodically by nurse or doctor. When the baby's head crowned, the doctor was called. The woman was wheeled to a brightly lit delivery room and positioned on her back on a metal delivery table, her legs raised into stirrups. The doctor, in surgical mask and gown, helped deliver the baby. After delivery, the baby went to the nursery, and the mother was wheeled to the recovery room, where she was checked to make sure the medication was wearing off properly and bleeding was not excessive. She would go to another room for postpartum care, until checkout two or three days later. Dividing birth into these stages was efficient for the hospital and ensured a certain standard of care at each step.

Some hospitals still follow this routine. But the demand for more family-centered, personalized maternity care has nudged many hospitals into regarding labor and delivery as one unbroken event, as it naturally occurs. Since the mid-1980s, many have changed their policies and redesigned their maternity wards to allow a less fragmented birth process. Many hospitals now have "birthing suites" or "LDR" rooms, which allow labor, delivery, and recovery all in one place. (Some, called LDRP rooms, include postpartum care.) The rooms are furnished to feel more like home than a hospital, although they usually fall in between, resembling a modest hotel room, decorated in pastel colors. The rooms generally have a birthing bed, which is a hospital bed that can be dismantled so that the foot of the bed is removed for delivery, and usually a private bath, some with an extra-large shower or a tub with whirlpool jets. A fetal monitor, resuscitation equipment, and bright lights are tucked away in a closet or wardrobe until needed.

Nurse-midwives like working in hospitals with birthing rooms because they make it easier to approach childbirth as a continuum. In fact, many nurse-midwives are former labor and delivery nurses who went to midwifery school because they wanted to help women through the whole experience of childbirth, not just one component. In a hospital that does not have birthing suites, nurse-midwives try to avoid the delivery room, and allow women to deliver in bed in the room where they labored, meaning a woman may have to switch rooms only once, for postpartum care. Long before anyone invented an LDRP or a birthing suite, nurse-midwives were helping women through labor and delivery all in one room. A birthing room can be created in any room by the attitude toward birth. It is not defined by the furniture and the wallpaper.

"MY BABY . . . MY BIRTH"

Because nurse-midwives allow a normal labor to proceed without interference, it is possible to have a completely natural childbirth in a hospital, as was the case for Nancy, whose labor and delivery were described at the beginning of Chapter 1. The Miami lawyer had absolutely no doubt she would give birth to Rebecca in a hospital—that was the only place that seemed safe to her. But she wanted to be in control. It was her body and her baby. She wanted to help decide what procedures would be done, and to set the tone for the birth. She wanted to have some say.

That feeling of involvement was missing with the birth of her first child. When she first became pregnant, she began prenatal care with her long-time OB/GYN whose fatherly "don't worry, I'll take care of it" approach made her feel secure in her teens and twenties. As the months of her first pregnancy wore on, that relationship seemed awkward. She was a grown and accomplished woman, about to become a mother. The notion that someone else would "take care of" this momentous passage in her life struck her as odd. She wanted more input, more responsibility, more control.

During childbirth classes, Nancy heard about two nurse-midwives in private practice. After the birth, Nancy began going to them—Dianne Fabiszewski and Sharron O'Brien of Childbirth Associates, Inc.—for her yearly gynecological care. She felt so comfortable with the nurse-midwives, she looked forward to having her next baby with them. When a pregnancy test came back positive, their hugs and enthusiasm set the stage for the joyful pregnancy and birth ahead.

To her family and friends, "midwife" sounded risky, even though Nancy explained that nurse-midwives accept only the healthiest women, that she would be having the baby in a hospital, that birth generally was an uncomplicated event.

"People said to me, 'You could afford anything, you could afford to fly a doctor in. Why would you go to a midwife?' " Nancy said. "People might have expected that if I were more earthy, but people don't perceive me that way."

Instinctively, though, Nancy knew the decision was right for her. She believed in herself, and her ability to choose what would be best for her and her baby. And she knew the nurse-midwives supported her way of thinking.

"My feeling was, 'I want to be in control.' This is my body, this is my birth, this is probably my last child. I wanted to really be in touch with it," she said. "I wanted to be involved in the decision and the management of it. And I wanted it to be my birth, and I wanted support for that. I wanted to do it in a way that was taking the least amount of risk as I possibly could in giving birth, but I wanted to be in control."

Her husband Donald agreed the decision was hers, and supported her choice. Still, he cautioned her that with such high expectations for the birth she was bound to be disappointed. She shouldn't expect everything to go perfectly. But in the end, Nancy's experience was better than even she had hoped for.

That's not to say delivering a baby is easy, although her labor started out that way. Twice during her fortieth week, contractions started and stopped. Then, after dawn on her due date, contractions began coming at regular seven-minute intervals. At 7 a.m. Nancy called Dianne, who told her to eat breakfast and call Donald, who had just left for work. Dianne would meet them at the hospital at 9:30 a.m. Nancy's mother came over to stay with three-year-old Rachel.

When Nancy and Donald arrived at the hospital, all the birthing rooms were occupied, so they settled into another room. Contractions barely interrupted Nancy's conversation or movement, and Dianne warned her this still could be false labor or very early labor. But when they moved into a birthing room a few minutes later and Dianne did the internal exam, Nancy was six centimeters dilated. There certainly would be a baby that day!

Dianne ordered a second breakfast for Nancy, to make sure she would have energy for the work ahead. Wearing a flowered kimono over her hospital gown, Nancy unpacked her bag, then walked the hospital halls with Donald, while Dianne attended to some other business nearby.

By noon, the contractions were closer together, but still very manageable to Nancy. She ate the turkey sandwich she had packed. The next internal exam showed that Nancy was dilated almost eight centimeters. Dianne offered to break her bag of waters to prod labor into the home stretch but Nancy said no. She felt comfortable with the natural course of her labor and saw no reason to tamper with it. "I thought it was going well, I just wanted to let it progress," she said.

With her favorite tapes playing in the background, Nancy settled into a rocking chair. Dianne sat by her, and they chatted about whatever came to mind—decisions in their lives, balancing a career with family. When a contraction came, Dianne breathed with her. Then they picked up the conversation.

By about 2 p.m., a wave of nausea made Nancy wonder whether the turkey sandwich was such a good idea after all. It made no difference, Dianne assured her: with or without food, many women feel nausea by that point in labor. At least the snack would give her energy for pushing. By 4 p.m. Nancy was completely dilated and two labor nurses came in to help. They removed the bottom portion of the birthing bed, and brought a lamp to warm the baby. Dianne asked again if Nancy wanted her water broken; again Nancy declined. She climbed into bed and adjusted it between lying and sitting. Dianne suggested Nancy phone her mother and Rachel to tell them that the baby was on its way. Then Nancy felt an urge to push. She asked Dianne to break the bag of waters.

That final half hour was the worst part. Nancy moaned through each contraction, pushing downward. Donald helped her regain composure between contractions, breathing with her as Vivaldi's *Four Seasons* played quietly. But as the pushing got more painful, Nancy started to panic. "Do something to get this baby out!" she told

Dianne. Dianne said she would cut a small episiotomy.
For the next few pushes, a nurse supported one knee and
Donald held the other. Then from the foot of the bed,
Donald said the baby was crowning. Nancy reached
down—and touched her baby's head!

"Slow, slow," Dianne coached as Nancy moaned with
the next-to-last push. Only eighteen minutes after Nancy
began pushing, the head was born. Dianne eased out one
shoulder, then the next. Then Donald took over, lifting
his squalling, healthy daughter onto his wife's belly.

With her first birth, Nancy's mind was fogged by Demerol, and she could not concentrate. As the baby
crowned, Nancy had been shuttled from the labor to delivery room and received a second dose of epidural anesthesia to numb her for the delivery. Then her doctor was
called away for an emergency, and the baby moved back
up the birth canal because anesthesia masked her urge to
push. After the birth, Nancy was frustrated by the many
obstacles between her and her baby. Yearning for contact
with her baby on the first night, Nancy found herself
standing outside the nursery and watching her tiny
daughter for an hour, unable to hold her because it was
not the scheduled feeding time.

With her second birth, Nancy knew she did not want
to be separated from her baby, and she never was. From
the moment of birth, Nancy held her skin-to-skin, and
nursed her immediately. Donald covered the newborn with
a warmed receiving blanket and caressed his new daughter's legs and arms to welcome her into the world. Dianne
clamped the cord and Donald cut it. The baby stayed right
on Nancy's belly as Dianne and the nurse cleaned the infant, took her footprints, and put on her identification
bracelet.

What Nancy especially liked was the way Dianne stayed
with her and Rebecca after the birth. She did not just sew

up Nancy's cut and leave. She played with the baby as the neonatologist examined her. She grimaced along with Nancy when the baby's heel was pricked for the phenyl-ketonuria (PKU) blood test.

"She wasn't just a medical technician," Nancy said. "She was really there for me. She was really there for the family. That meant a lot that she was so sincerely involved with us."

Within an hour of the birth, other family members arrived. Rachel hugged her mother, and shyly touched her tiny new sister. Grandparents held the baby and remarked on the family resemblance. Nancy loved having everyone so close together, and loved how she could be with her baby the whole time.

"This was really my birth," she said. "I was the one who got to stay with the baby, and not all the nurses taking her away and doing all these things."

Wide awake from the unmedicated birth, it was a few hours after the birth that pain relief crossed Nancy's mind for the first time that day. She took two Tylenol for her afterpains and achiness. The next day, Dianne came back to check on Nancy and to talk about whatever was on her mind. Nancy said she was mortified by the noises she made at the end of labor, at her loss of control, at the way she ordered Dianne to "do something" near the end. The nurse-midwife laughed and reassured her that in childbirth, there is no such thing as embarrassment.

"What do you expect?" Dianne said. "You delivered a baby. You were wonderful, you were unbelievable."

Deep down, Nancy felt that way too. For all but a few panicky seconds, Nancy felt very much that she was the power behind this birth. *She* was giving birth to this baby. She was aware of every contraction and every sensation, completely in touch with the amazing and powerful process of bringing forth a child. She was very proud of how Rebecca came into the world—in the peaceful, loving way that seemed right to her. It was a wonderful start, she thought, for mother and daughter.

ADVANTAGES OF HOSPITAL BIRTH

Safety is the primary reason most women choose a hospital for a nurse-midwife birth. Another is that with some nurse-midwives who work in hospitals, you may not have to switch entirely to the care of the doctor if a complication develops; the nurse-midwife and her consulting physician may co-manage.

Other advantages become apparent after the baby is born. Laura, who spent so little time in the hospital before the birth described in Chapter 3, found her two-day hospital stay afterward to be a well-deserved rest. As she put it: "After all that work, who wants to clean up?" Stitches and general soreness made it hard for her to get around at first. She was glad to have complete meals brought to her. She liked being in a bed that she did not have to *think* about making. And it was reassuring to have someone check on her daily.

If you have small children at home, the time in the hospital may be especially welcome. Even if you have an extremely helpful husband, mother, or professional help waiting for you at home, inevitably your other children will place demands on your energy and attention. Although some mothers prefer to be home as soon as possible after birth, others find the day or two in the hospital to be a time to rest from the work of delivery before beginning a new marathon at home.

Even if you choose to have your baby room-in with you in the hospital, the nurses will take the newborn to the nursery for a few hours if you like. Some mothers, particularly first-timers, find themselves so excited or nervous about the newborn, they cannot sleep much when the baby is with them at first. In the hospital, your nurse-midwife or other nurses are available to help you with breastfeeding, bathing your child and other babycare. A pediatrician examines the baby right in the hospital, saving you the trip during the first week after birth.

A CONSTANT PRESENCE, A CALM VOICE

Karen, from Brooklyn, spent nearly three days in early labor at home with her second child. When her bag of waters finally broke, her nurse-midwife admitted her to the hospital. But in the next few hours, she dilated little. The nurse-midwife hooked up the electronic fetal monitor; after a while, the baby's heart-rate plummeted. The nurse-midwife immediately called the doctor, and gave Karen oxygen. Karen would need what she called "all that high-tech nonsense" after all.

Within minutes, the nurse-midwife and Karen were on the way to the operating room, where the doctor was preparing for a cesarean delivery. All the while, Karen felt little panic—to her own surprise. Once it was clear she was going to have a cesarean, there was little that midwife or mother could do. Meanwhile the presence of her nurse-midwife was a huge comfort during what could have been a very frightening time. The midwife's soothing voice made the difference for Karen, a voice that did not leave her side.

"It was the midwife's words, very calm, that made me feel better," she said. "I felt that everything was under control."

The reason for the slow labor, and then the dropped heart rate, was that the baby was positioned oddly, not straight down into the birth canal. There was no way to know that until the cesarean. But as soon as the baby showed signs of distress, the nurse-midwife knew the doctor should be called. Then she stayed right by Karen, through the cesarean until after she could see that both Karen and healthy little Eden were going to be fine.

CYBILL SHEPHERD—IT'S A GIRL! AND A BOY!

Like so many other mothers, Cybill Shepherd describes nurse-midwife birth in a hospital as "the best of everything."

"It's the best thing for you and the best thing for your baby," she says. "You always have the doctor right there and all the emergency things. You don't have to travel somewhere for backup, which you probably won't need. And you have less chance of needing it with a nurse-midwife."

When Cybill became pregnant with twins eight years after the birth of her daughter, she was dismayed to find that nurse-midwives usually do not handle twins. Although twins usually are delivered by cesarean birth in the United States, she shopped until she found a Los Angeles doctor who would let her try to deliver vaginally. He also agreed that two nurse-midwives could be present at the birth to assist her in labor and delivery. He would stand aside, as long as there were no complications. Labor lasted thirteen hours—a difficult time for Cybill, but she had the support she wanted and needed.

"The nurse-midwives stayed in my face with breathing and helping me," she said. "They helped me walk around and gave me enormous support."

The first twin born, Ariel, was a normal head-first delivery into the hands of nurse-midwives. But as Ariel moved through the birth canal, she pushed her twin brother sideways. That's when the doctor got involved. Aware that the complication could call for an immediate cesarean, the doctor, nurse-midwives, and an obstetrical nurse all helped, using their hands, to turn the baby. Zach turned head down and was delivered vaginally six minutes after his sister.

"The doctor's training is not to help women through labor; it is to be prepared for complications," Cybill said. "He did his job brilliantly."

Cybill was extremely grateful to have such skilled professionals, who also took into account her desires. They helped her give birth in a way that left her feeling proud and satisfied.

"It was my greatest sense of accomplishment in my life, that feeling after giving birth to twins," she said.

"To have what you want at your birth, that's the safest thing for you and your baby. It allows you to take control so that in that moment of birth when you must lose control, when it's so difficult, you are surrounded by people who can support you not only physically but mentally and emotionally. They almost breathe for you, to keep you breathing."

THE NURSE-MIDWIFE DIFFERENCE

In a hospital, a nurse-midwife helps make the experience as personal and non-institutional as possible. One way is by using high-tech options only if needed, rather than routinely. Also, women who give birth with nurse-midwives spend less time in the hospital—coming late in labor after phone contact in the early hours, and being discharged as soon as six hours after birth if all is well and the mother feels ready. Both of these factors reiterate the message that childbirth is not an illness. And, both factors add up to smaller hospital bills. More particulars on the cost of nurse-midwifery care are explained in Chapter 11.

Nurse-midwives also tend to involve the birth partner more than physicians do—reading the electronic fetal monitor, if one is being used; massaging during contractions; providing physical support for the pushing stage. And, of course, the father may be the first to hold his baby.

The most significant difference between hospital birth with a nurse-midwife and with a doctor is the personalized support and encouragement, in ways you may not anticipate. When choosing care, many first-time mothers are so absorbed in the details of pregnancy, they do not focus on the particulars of the birth until the six or seventh month. But these details can shape an experience that will be with you for the rest of your life. Here are a few things to be aware of as you choose your care:

Familiarity: If you are in a physician's care, the doctor you become accustomed to during prenatal care probably will not be the person to first examine you when you arrive in labor. You will be admitted and checked by nurses or doctors (often residents) you have never met. You may see your own doctor, or a partner in the same practice, only briefly while you are in labor. He or she will return when you begin pushing, or soon after.

Consistency: Depending on the policy and staff-to-patient ratio at the hospital, the labor nurse assigned to you may stay with you the whole time or shuttle between a number of laboring women. When the shift changes, so will nurses and residents. That can be unsettling. Also, having different people checking you may lead to inconsistent measures of your progress. Such inconsistency may suggest you are not progressing. A nurse-midwife who stays by your side through much of labor is usually the only one examining your cervix. She has a feel for your particular labor and can tell more quickly if it is deviating from normal.

Predictability: Surprises are the last thing you want as you try to cope with labor. But you may find that agreements made with your doctor in prenatal care, such as no IV unless indicated, do not hold with nurses who insist on following standard hospital procedures unless the doctor left other instructions in your chart. And if one of the doctor's partners is on call for your labor, your prior agreements may not be honored. For instance, your doctor may feel comfortable delivering a baby in a birthing room, but a colleague may insist on the delivery room.

Midwifery has different meanings to different midwives. Some purists say that the bustle of a hospital rules out "true" practice of midwifery. Regardless, hospital birth is the option with which many women and nurse-midwives are most comfortable. For women who require a hospital for medical reasons or safety concerns, a nurse-midwife helps avoid unnecessary intervention and provides personal support.

DENISE'S STORY

Denise, the hospital social worker and mother from outside Detroit, learned from two births in the same hospital the difference a nurse-midwife can make. Early in her first pregnancy, she developed hypertension, forcing her to switch from a nurse-midwife to a doctor. With the second pregnancy, her blood pressure stayed in a normal range until the very end. The doctor and nurse-midwife decided the nurse-midwife could supervise the labor. High blood pressure can be dangerous in labor because of possible complications if the baby does not get enough oxygen. Denise felt that the nurse-midwife's vigilance and supervision of her medical problems minimized the risks of her condition while allowing her the kind of birth experience she wanted.

Both times labor was induced because of the hypertension. A laboring woman with hypertension is encouraged to lie on her left side, to accelerate blood flow to the baby. With the first baby, Denise's physician told her simply not to move from that position once labor began so as not to endanger the baby. After Pitocin was given she was left largely on her own, monitored occasionally by nurses. Denise found, however, that spending hours in one position is a painful addition to the discomforts of labor. With the second baby, Denise's nurse-midwife did not require Denise to stay on her side the whole time. Instead, she let Denise move around, but monitored her blood pressure and the baby's heartbeat almost constantly.

"You just can't imagine the difference being allowed to sit up and change positions between contractions," Denise said. "She didn't have to worry about me getting in trouble because she wasn't going out the door. She knew if I was getting in any trouble and she would get me back into position on my side. There was no risk to me or the baby because the midwife was there. . . . She could do the little extra things that couldn't have been done with the first baby."

The midwife offered sips of orange juice throughout active labor, which surprised Denise. In her previous labor she was allowed only ice chips in case she needed emergency surgery. But her nurse-midwife thought the boost would help her *avoid* a cesarean.

"I took the sips of orange juice, it gave me so much additional energy. It's little things that mean so much," Denise said. "Being allowed to have a couple sips of orange juice make all the difference in the world to keep you going. And you are so much more comfortable during labor because of that."

That presence of her nurse-midwife was the most crucial difference between the two births.

"She was there for me," Denise said. "With the first baby, I did not know this resident, I didn't know the nurses. And they were the ones who were really there to deliver me.

"Whereas with my second delivery, Thersa [the nurse-midwife] was there from the moment I began to be induced to the delivery. It's a whole different feeling of security. It felt like having a friend there with you."

"My husband was excellent. But it was very nice to have someone there who totally understood the medical situation in addition. Having the two of them was ideal."

ENHANCING THE EXPERIENCE

Jane, the New York lawyer who interviewed six obstetricians and three nurse-midwife teams before choosing a nurse-midwife, knew she was not a candidate for out-of-hospital birth. She had confidence in her body and expected a natural birth, without medication or intravenous, but she wanted to be in a hospital just in case. She was comfortable in hospitals and confident in them, having accompanied her father, a surgeon, on Saturday morning rounds when she was a child.

By the time Jane's labor was far enough along for admission to the hospital early on a Tuesday morning, she already had been having contractions at home since Sunday. Exhausted from more than forty-eight hours of early labor, Jane and her nurse-midwife agreed that Demerol was a good idea. The drug did not bring much pain relief, but it helped Jane sleep between contractions, sometimes as long as twenty minutes. Her nurse-midwife never left her room.

By noon, however, Jane felt overwhelmed by each

contraction. She was afraid she could not tolerate the rest of labor and asked for an epidural. At the same time, her nurse-midwife was concerned that Jane was dilating very slowly for someone who had been in labor so long. She suggested Pitocin. Jane and her husband agreed. The doctor arrived and agreed with those decisions.

Immediately after the anesthesiologist gave the epidural, Jane felt better. The relief from pain invigorated her. Drugs, anesthesia, and an IV were not part of the birth she had imagined, but in view of her slow labor, she felt she was taking the best options.

"I trusted the midwives and knew they would do these things only because they were necessary," she said. "I knew they were doing it not because it was routine but because it was best."

Afterward, she could not imagine the experience without the nurse-midwife. The presence of her husband was a comfort, certainly, but it was the support of her nurse-midwife—the skills, knowledge and experience—that made the real difference.

"She was there. The hand-holding was tremendous," Jane said. "I wasn't coherent to have a conversation with my husband. His presence was nice. Hers was tremendous."

When contractions became more difficult, Jane's confidence melted into "blind fear." The midwife and doctor had let the epidural wear off so that Jane would feel the urge to push. And she felt it, sure enough. During those last few minutes, the pain was so intense, Jane scarcely was aware of her surroundings. She clenched her eyes shut, and concentrated, retreating into her own world. Then she heard the voice of her midwife: "Open your eyes Jane, you're going to miss everything."

Jane opened her eyes and saw a miracle.

"I couldn't believe this baby was coming out of me," Jane said. "All my life I will remember it. Had my midwife not told me to open my eyes, I never would have seen it."

HOSPITALS ARE NOT FOR EVERYONE

Despite the advantages of hospital birth, some people are bothered by the rules, room sharing, noise, and lack of privacy that may be part of a hospital stay. And some hospitals have policies that clash with the ideal practice of nurse-midwifery. For instance, nurse-midwives do not automatically regard meconium (fecal matter) in the amniotic fluid as a sign of fetal distress; they consider the fluid's color and other factors. Yet in some hospitals, the presence of meconium requires that the birth take place in a delivery room with resuscitation equipment rather than in a birthing room.

There also may be intrusions. During the first few hours after Roi gave birth to her daughter she wanted to be alone with her baby and her husband. They paid extra for a private room, so they could be together quietly as a family. They felt bothered by what seemed like an incessant and needless parade of people into the room. A photographer, a hospital worker talking about programs for new mothers, and a breastfeeding instructor—although Roi and baby were managing fine—all came in uninvited.

"They were a little insensitive to what it's like to have a newborn, which is a little peculiar, since that's their job," Roi said.

Hospitals also may not be best if you want to have your other children present at the birth. Some hospitals do not allow it. Others do, but a hospital is a boring and confining place for a child during the long hours of labor.

SHOPPING FOR A HOSPITAL

Before you sign on with a nurse-midwife who does hospital births, tour the maternity ward where women in her care deliver to see if the arrangement suits you. A nurse-midwife generally works in one hospital only. If you are comparing a number of nurse-midwives (and doctors), the various settings may factor into your decision. Once labor is underway, women find the people more significant than the surroundings, but you will feel better going into labor if you have chosen a place you like. Here are questions to ask yourself, the nurse-midwife, and the hospital staff as you make your decision.

Is surgery, that is—a cesarean—immediately available?
Are specialists on-duty in the hospital around the clock?
Is there an intensive care unit for newborns?

Many people assume that all hospitals have the same degree of services available, but they do not. Not all have a complete array of medical specialists on duty at all times, including the anesthesiologist and obstetrician necessary for a cesarean section. Only those rated for tertiary care, usually in big cities or university affiliated, are staffed and equipped for extreme emergencies and illnesses around the clock. These hospitals generally have a neonatal intensive care unit, an anesthesiologist, obstetrician, neonatologist, and perinatologist immediately available. Smaller community hospitals may have some of these special services; others may not have an obstetrician, or even a physician, in the hospital at all times. Know what kind of hospital you are going to, how long it would take to prepare for a cesarean and how far you must travel if your baby needs to be transferred to a neonatal intensive care unit.

What is the room like? Will I be comfortable here?

Ask whether you will be sharing a room with someone, whether private rooms cost extra, and whether you
will have your own bathroom. Does the room have a
shower or tub big enough for a very pregnant woman?
Curtains and wallpaper look nice, but at the time of labor
you will be more concerned about privacy, comfort, and
convenience.

*If there are birthing suites, is one usually available? Or,
are they frequently in use?*

Do not assume you definitely will have your baby in
the room you see on the hospital tour. In some hospitals,
a birthing suite is usually available to any woman who
wants one. But some hospitals have only one or two
birthing suites, while twenty maternity patients are in the
hospital all at once. Given the unpredictability of labor,
rooms are on a first come, first served basis. Ask the hospital staff and the nurse-midwives whether women arriving in labor often find the rooms already occupied. On
the other hand, if doctors at a hospital have been slow to
break delivery room habits, you may find the birthing
rooms almost always empty.

Are there places to walk during labor?

Depending on the progress of your labor, you may have
a lot of time on your hands after you arrive. If the hospital is far from your home, you may arrive early for an
internal exam and be told to go for a walk rather than be
admitted right away. Are there pleasant places to walk—
a nearby park or shopping mall?

*What family members are allowed into my room, and
when? May fathers stay overnight?*

Is a friend or relative permitted to be with you, in addition to your husband or partner, during labor? Are there

specific visiting hours for grandparents and other children? Some birthing rooms are equipped with comfy lounge chairs or couches for partners who want to spend the night. Other hospitals do not permit fathers to stay.

What is the hospital's routine for the baby after birth? Is rooming-in allowed?

Hospitals where nurse-midwives work almost always permit the baby to remain in the room with the mother. Even if the hospital's standard policy is to whisk the baby off to the nursery, the rule may be bent for women in the care of nurse-midwives. But you will still want to know what procedures the hospital follows for eye drops, bathing, treating jaundice, and feeding. If your baby spends time in the nursery and you are breastfeeding, your nurse-midwife will help arrange with the nurses not to bottle-feed sugar water to your baby, which would disrupt the baby's appetite.

Your nurse-midwife also is available to help you decide whether you want a male baby to be circumcised; some nurse-midwives perform the procedure.

When will my baby and I be discharged?

Under a doctor's care, most women stay in the hospital one to two days after vaginal birth and three to five days after cesarean. Some nurse-midwives allow mother and baby to go home as soon as six hours after birth if both are healthy. The time of discharge may depend on hospital policy; some hospitals do not allow discharge sooner than twenty-four hours after birth.

What rules must I follow?

Some hospitals allow you to wear only hospital-issue clothing, forbid food during labor, and restrict visiting hours even for the patients of nurse-midwives. Ask about these rules in advance, so you will not be surprised.

What is the relationship of the nurse-midwife or nurse-midwives with the hospital staff?

The rapport of your nurse-midwife with doctors and nurses in the hospital is crucial. You want to know that if there is a complication your nurse-midwife will have the complete cooperation and trust of the consulting physician and any other specialists and nurses in the hospital. In some hospitals, particularly those owned by HMOs or in a university system, nurse-midwives are part of the health-care team for the majority of births and are fully accepted and integrated into the hospital. In a handful of hospitals, however, particularly where nurse-midwives are new or few in number, they are viewed warily. Nurses and doctors may resent a nurse-midwife's autonomy and deviation from hospital protocol. If you can avoid this situation, you should.

Fortunately, in many hospitals the opposite is true. Maternity nurses, residents, and other doctors like the nurse-midwife style of care so much they take extra pains to continue the personal, family-centered approach. That is the hospital to look for.

During a hospital tour ask yourself if you could be comfortable there, if you feel good about having your baby there. If the answer is no, you may want to keep looking for another hospital, and possibly another nurse-midwife. Some women who start out thinking they want a hospital birth find hospital regulations too confining. For them, a birth center or home birth may be more suitable.

9.

BIRTH CENTERS

*"Going to a hospital seemed so foreign to my
whole way of thinking, especially for what
seemed like a healthy experience. . . . I really
had the feeling that it was a privilege to give birth
and I didn't want to miss it."*
—*BRENDA, A FIRST-TIME MOTHER*

WHEN BRENDA BECAME pregnant with her first child, she
wanted care that fit with what she called her "healthy
frame of mind." Her gynecologist did not handle obstetrics. She met with an obstetrician, but felt he was too
quick to do cesareans. The twenty-six-year-old book de-
signer from Los Angeles began looking into alternatives.
To her way of thinking, a normal, healthy birth was a
joyful occasion, one that did not fit with the sickness and
high-tech gadgetry of a hospital. At the other end of the
spectrum, she knew some women had their babies at
home, but as a first-time mother, she was too nervous to
consider that. A birth center sounded right for her.

At the first center she visited, she liked the approach,
but she was a little uneasy. When she asked questions, the
answers seemed skimpy. And the decor was just not her

style. As an artist, Brenda felt a strong reaction to visual things around her. The antique furniture that some mothers love seemed "old ladyish" to her. She knew she just would not be comfortable there.

The next center was an entirely different story. Right away she felt comfortable. By the time the orientation and tour were over at the Natural Childbirth Institute and Women's Health Center in Culver City, she knew "hands down, no question, that's where I would have my baby." She liked the nurse-midwife's upfront approach. The orientation alone made her feel more confident about her own ability to nurture and deliver a healthy baby.

Brenda came to her prenatal visits at the center with a full page of questions. The nurse-midwives encouraged the interest she was taking in her pregnancy. At each visit, weighing herself and testing her own urine made her feel even more connected to her body and her baby. The more she learned about pregnancy and birth, the fewer her fears.

She definitely felt the center was the best place for her to have her baby, but two nagging concerns stayed with her from that first orientation visit. The first was pain medication. Some birth centers make pain medication available, but not this one.

"I didn't want to use drugs. But I'd never had a baby before," Brenda worried. "What if it was intensely horrible and I couldn't stand it? I wanted to have an out."

The center's outlook was that the availability of medication distracts a mother and makes her more likely to use it at a time when she should focus on birthing her baby. In theory, Brenda agreed; in reality, she was afraid. The nurse-midwife listened to her fears. She agreed that birth would be painful, but said a relaxing and supportive environment would help make the pain manageable. Brenda still had some trepidation, but the midwife's acknowledgment of her fears somehow comforted her.

Her other concern was going home the same day as the

birth, which is the center's policy. In just those few hours, how would she know how to take care of her baby? The nurse-midwife sensed her apprehension.

"She called me on it," Brenda said. "She said I would have to learn to care for my baby sooner or later, whether it was two hours after the birth or two weeks."

When those first labor pains came, Brenda still had concerns typical of almost every first-time mother, but with each new bit of knowledge and support, most of her fears had diminished. The birth would be with professionals she trusted, in a place she felt comfortable. Everyone there, she knew, shared with her and her husband the goal of a safe, natural, and peaceful transition for their baby from her womb into the world.

WHAT BIRTH CENTERS ARE, WHAT THEY ARE NOT

Birth centers are places where healthy pregnant women receive prenatal care and deliver their babies, with assistance. They offer the time and place for unhurried, low-tech birth guided by professionals with a standard for safety. Having a baby in a birth center is an experience families cherish because it allows for a peaceful, personal birth in a professional environment. Parents often feel very attached to their center, looking back on it as a loving place that enabled them to give their baby a start that was uniquely their own.

Specific options and services vary from one center to the next, although all strive to offer a homelike, affordable, and supportive environment for the birth itself. They generally include a private bedroom with a non-hospital double bed, homelike furnishings, soft lighting, and a private bath with an extra-wide shower or tub, often with whirlpool jets. A kitchen is usually available, and families bring their own food and drink for labor and for a celebration after the birth. Friends, grandparents, and children (with supervision) are all welcome at the birth.

Births take place with minimal intervention. Some medical equipment is available, however, to initiate treatment as needed: intravenous lines and fluids, oxygen for mother and baby, infant resuscitator, infant warmer, local anesthesia for use when repairing tears and episiotomies, and synthetic oxytocin to control postpartum bleeding. Some centers also have analgesic pain medication available but seldom use it.

Despite the medical equipment, birth centers are not mini-hospitals. They depend on the hospital with which they are affiliated and do not duplicate a hospital's technology. They do not perform cesareans; they do not offer the services of an anesthesiologist, which means no epidurals; they do not have intensive care units for mothers or newborns; they do not transfuse blood. They do not induce labor with drugs, and very few use electronic fetal monitors. They do not provide meals or newborn nursery care.

Nurse-midwives in birth centers maintain strong safety records by accepting only women whose good health makes them least likely to have complications and often have more stringent criteria than those who attend hospital births. Standards for accepting women vary among centers, as do guidelines for conditions requiring transfer out of the center's care. Every center must have a consulting physician who accepts transfers during pregnancy and labor. It is important for a center to have a good working relationship with a nearby hospital that will accept a woman in labor who develops a complication.

Most birth centers are free-standing, unattached to any other building or institution; a few are attached to hospitals. Most are owned by nurse-midwives or doctors; a smaller number are not-for-profit centers governed by a board of directors. In most, but not all, nurse-midwives provide most of the care and attend the births. Prenatal visits take place in the center, and by the time of the birth the surroundings are familiar to the whole family.

MEETING A NEED

Out-of-hospital birth centers represent a new generation of health care. In order to meet the desires of families to have control over their births, away from the medical model of care, a free-standing birth center opened in New York City in 1975. The Childbearing Center, as it is still called, was launched by the Maternity Center Association, the private, nonprofit agency that had opened the country's first nurse-midwifery school four decades earlier. In the early 1970s, Maternity Center officials were hearing that more and more couples around the country were resorting to unattended home births because they did not like what hospitals offered. The Maternity Center listened to families' complaints and responded with a plan that combined the best of medical science with the needs of families for privacy, personal attention, closeness, and celebration. The resulting birth center, in a large house on Manhattan's Upper East Side, opened with approval from the New York State Department of Health. Since 1975, nearly four thousand babies have been born there.

Other centers followed. In 1983, the Maternity Center Association established the National Association of Childbearing Centers to share information and set standards for safe operation. By the early 1990s, there were about 135 free-standing birth centers in 37 states.

Centers are regulated in two ways. The first is state licensure. In thirty states, free-standing birth centers have their own licensing category and cannot operate unless they meet criteria set down by the state. The second type of regulation is voluntary accreditation by the Commission for the Accreditation of Freestanding Birth Centers. Since the late 1980s this agency has provided a professional stamp of approval for centers that meet its standards for safety, services, and sound management. By 1992, twenty centers had received accreditation and a dozen others were in the process.

Most women choose the centers for their approach to birth, while other clients are attracted by the affordable cost—about half that of a regular hospital stay—along with the birth-center philosophy. Some birth-center models were developed in the migrant health system, notably one that opened in Raymondville, Texas, in 1972, to meet the needs of people receiving government subsidies. That center was so successful that government officials sought to duplicate it elsewhere. A successful urban model of care is in the Bronx in New York, where the Maternity Center Association opened the Childbearing Center of Morris Heights in 1988, created primarily for low-income women in the surrounding neighborhoods. Within three years of the center's opening, neighborhood women who had given birth there were on the center's task force, helping to shape policies and new health programs there.

THE BIRTH CENTER EXPERIENCE

For Brenda and her husband David, the birth center surpassed their expectations, which is not to say the birth went like clockwork. Few births do. The first contraction came when Brenda was home alone, two days past her due date. David was having a final night out with a buddy before facing fatherhood. Just as Brenda finished a midnight lullaby to the baby in her belly, she felt what she thought was a slight contraction. Then another. She was excited, but knew she should go to sleep. Such mild contractions meant the birth was still many hours away.

At 6 a.m., a contraction woke her—a little stronger than the ones she felt earlier. Then to her delight, the mucus plug came out—this was labor for certain! She called her nurse-midwife and woke David. So far, the contractions were "a piece of cake," but as the day wore on, it was hard work to keep labor going. The contractions were three minutes apart, but still weak and only thirty seconds long. Brenda thought if she kept active, she could move the labor along. Her nurse-midwife suggested a swim, or a walk. Swimming felt terrific. Then when she and David were well into a long, brisk walk the contractions abruptly strengthened. The couple walked back slowly and climbed into the car for the birth center.

An internal exam by one of the center's nurse-midwives and its owner, Nancy McNeese, showed Brenda was dilated about three centimeters. It was about 7 p.m. Nancy suggested another walk, on the beach nearby, but with the next contraction, Brenda doubled over. It was time to stay put.

From then on, Brenda said, labor "was hard, hard work." She spent most of the time in the birth center's hot tub, which felt much better to her than being in bed and soothed her painful back labor. The nurse-midwife encouraged her to try different positions to keep her labor moving along, which Brenda appreciated.

"It's such an intense experience to be in labor, you don't think that creatively," she said. "You don't think of trying different positions."

Although Brenda's description of labor is echoed by other birth center mothers, the actual birth was unusual. Brenda gave birth in the specially designed tub, an option provided at only a few birth centers in the U.S. Many centers and even hospitals have tubs where women spend some of their labor, but only a few have water births.

Toward the end of labor, the water felt so good, Brenda stayed in the tub. Months earlier, she had decided she wanted a water birth. But one of the nurse-midwives at the center had encouraged her to think "maybe" rather than "definitely"; many women change their minds once labor begins. When Brenda felt the urge to push, she wanted to stay in the tub; but she made little progress. Nancy suggested she try a different position outside the tub.

"Oh, that was so painful," Brenda said. "I got back in the tub. It was so much better in the water. I don't know how people do it otherwise. It's just so much better to have something else supporting you."

While Brenda floated in the tub with an inflatable pillow under her head, her husband crouched outside the tub and held one leg. Nancy was on the other side.

"I was barking out commands—put your hands there, harder!" Brenda remembered, with surprise at how insistent she became. "In retrospect, that felt really good that I was able to do that—just be completely into my body."

Soon enough, when Brenda reached down, she felt her baby's head. Nancy, her hands ready, caught 7-pound, 10-ounce Brian under the water.

"It felt great the moment he came out of me," Brenda said. "It was a wonderful feeling to have the baby slip out of me."

Nancy placed Brian right onto Brenda's chest. For twenty minutes, Brenda rested blissfully in the tub, her baby in her arms. He was alert, with eyes wide open.

"It was just really fabulous to be holding this baby," Brenda said. When it was time to deliver the placenta, Nancy helped Brenda into one of the homey birthing rooms and David took the baby. Meanwhile father and son were led to a separate room, and left alone together.

David was awed by the birth, but he felt distant from it. The birth and the baby were happening to Brenda, but were alien to him. As Brian was born, David saw the child still connected to Brenda, nourished by the umbilical cord and then by breast milk. But after cutting the umbilical cord and then sitting alone with the baby, David felt the purest of connections. This was *his* child. This tiny human being, with blue eyes fixed clearly on him, was dependent on him and would be part of his life forever. It was a wonderful bonding between father and son.

"He was just gazing at me with these beautiful blue eyes," David said. "He didn't squirm, he didn't cry. But he was very alert, very much alive. He liked being with me, and I liked being with him."

A few hours later, the new family was ready to go home. The concerns that had been so real for Brenda before the birth—no pain medication and going home so soon—did not matter. In fact, she would not have wanted the experience any other way.

Going through labor without pain medication made her hyperaware of her own body. Like many women who have unmedicated births, she described going deep inside her own body and having a near mystical experience.

"I stopped seeing clearly, but sound was very important," she said. "I was deep inside, but not altogether there."

It certainly hurt, as she expected, but pain was not the most lingering memory among the many sensations and emotions she felt. Bringing forth a new life indeed had been the privilege she envisioned. Brenda chose the birth center and water birth because she wanted to provide her baby with the easiest possible transition from the womb. Brian's alertness from the start and his good disposition during infancy she attributes partly to his gentle birth.

"The whole combination of having a natural, gradual transition and no drugs has to help," she said. "How can't it?"

Brenda also cherished going home with her newborn right away—"being home in my big bed with my little tiny baby." David took two weeks off from work to help out and so that his new family could get acquainted. It was a loving and peaceful time that flowed naturally from their experience at the birth center.

EACH CENTER IS DIFFERENT

All birth centers share the same general ethos, but there are significant differences from one center to the next in atmosphere, services, patient criteria, and who you see for care. As we've said, birth centers accept only healthy women, but their definitions of normal pregnancy differ slightly. Nearly all refuse women with high blood pressure, diabetes, cancer, heart disease, or other chronic illness. Some also rule out women who have had uterine surgery for fibroid removal or cesarean section; women dependent on medicine for asthma, thyroid condition, or mental illness; obese women, because it is hard to gauge the baby's growth and position; smokers; and women who have had five or more children, which increases the risk of postpartum hemorrhage.

There are some chronic health conditions, however, that do not disqualify a woman from care at most birth centers: RH negative blood, history of miscarriage, mitral valve prolapse, and other conditions that do not affect pregnancy. Some centers do vaginal birth after cesarean, but may require that the woman have had only one prior cesarean with a lower uterine cut.

Some centers have age criteria. The Childbearing Center in New York, for instance, takes no first-time mothers older than forty and no others older than forty-five. The Natural Childbirth Institute and Women's Health Center in Culver City, on the other hand, sets no age limit; a forty-three-year-old first-time mother safely delivered her baby there. If you are well into your pregnancy when you decide a birth center is what you want, you still may be able to enroll. Centers accept women up to 32 weeks, and sometimes as late as 36 weeks, with a good record of prenatal care.

Even after you have been accepted for care at a birth center, certain conditions may require that you transfer to an obstetrician's care and hospital birth. These include twins or other multiple births, placenta too close to the cervical opening, breech at term, or labor before 37 weeks or after 42 weeks. Gestational diabetes and pregnancy-related high blood pressure may also require transfer. All these conditions increase the likelihood of needing medical attention beyond the resources of a birth center.

VARIATIONS ON A THEME

From one center to the next, services vary. For instance, although almost all centers use tubs of warm water for pain relief and relaxation during labor, only a handful offer the water birth that Brenda had, an option that is new and controversial. Childbirth classes are required by most centers, but not all offer classes on the premises. The Maternity Center in Bethesda does not have its own childbirth class, but it provides all mothers with a baby care and breastfeeding "survival class" to prepare them to go home right after birth. Many centers also offer sibling classes, to prepare children for the birth of a new brother or sister. Some offer circumcision.

As with nurse-midwives in any birth setting, those in birth centers work collaboratively with a consulting physician—who rarely works within the birth center—to whom they refer women when complications arise in pregnancy or labor. Some states require one or two physician visits during pregnancy so that the physician can check the woman and they can meet each other; others leave it up to nurse-midwife or mother. New Jersey, for instance, requires all women to be seen twice by a doctor during pregnancy.

A woman who develops complications during pregnancy transfers to an obstetrician of her choice or one who has a working agreement with the center. If a complication develops during labor at the center, the nurse-midwives follow a prearranged protocol with their consulting physician. Usually that means calling the doctor and driving the woman to the hospital where the doctor admits her and takes over her care. Most complications are nonemergency and do not require an ambulance. At a few birth centers nurse-midwives have hospital privileges to admit and treat patients. For more on how complications during labor are handled, see the section on transfers, page 195.

Newborn and follow-up care varies from center to center. Nurse-midwives evaluate and examine the newborn; they administer the antibiotic eye ointment required in most states and the vitamin K injection to help blood clotting. A few centers also provide a pediatrician to check the baby immediately after birth, while other centers never use a pediatrician unless there is a problem. In a few centers, a pediatric nurse-practitioner makes the check. At the Childbearing Center in New York, all babies are seen by a pediatrician before going home; mother and baby are visited at home by a nurse the next day, a frequent service of birth centers. At the Maternity Center in Bethesda, on the other hand, the nurse-midwife does the initial evaluation and exam and parents take the newborn to a pediatrician within the next couple of days. The Women's Center of Martin County, Florida, phones mothers at home the day after the birth; mothers and babies return to the center two or three days later to remove the umbilical cord clamp, do the PKU blood test and complete the birth certificate. Two weeks later, a nurse-midwife visits mother and baby at home. Most centers offer a postpartum visit four to six weeks after birth and care between pregnancies, including Pap smear and birth control if desired.

PAIN MEDICATION

Pain medication is another variable. The Los Angeles birth center where Brenda had her baby uses none. That choice is not based on any principle that pain medication is bad or wrong—the nurse-midwives there simply regard medication as a form of medical intervention that may lead to complications and is more suitable for use in a hospital.

"Nancy [the center's owner] and I feel that pain medication alters the way the mother's uterus acts," nurse-midwife Susan Melnikow said. "The baby is affected as well. A birth center isn't the right place for that. That should be in a hospital."

But at the Women's Center of Martin County, just a block from a hospital, pain medication is available. Women should not think that just because it is a birth center, "you walk through the door and are handed a silver bullet to bite," one of the nurse-midwives explains at orientation. If you want an epidural, however, you should not be there, she explains. That is regional anesthesia and is done only in a hospital.

The Childbearing Center in New York used to keep Demerol on hand, but so rarely did women ask for it that the medicine usually expired and was discarded before it was used. The center stopped stocking it. In an environment of calm, trust, and realistic expectations, women find themselves able to endure the pain. It sounds simplistic when midwives say that the best medication in childbirth is love and support, but woman after woman has learned that is true.

BIRTH CENTERS PROMOTE CHOICES, RESPONSIBILITY

Birth centers promote confidence through education and shared responsibility. In response to the desires of women to learn about their bodies and be part of decisions, many centers encourage participation in prenatal care. Women take their own blood pressure, test their urine, and learn to understand their chart. This knowledge helps women feel confident in their choices, about birth and the important job of caring for a newborn. The emphasis on self-care may be greater in birth centers than in hospitals. With limited emergency equipment available, nurse-midwives at birth centers expect each mother to be as healthy as possible when labor begins. This may mean more stringent expectations for proper diet and exercise and avoidance of unhealthy habits, including smoking. Women are expected to prepare themselves for the birth physically, mentally, and emotionally.

At the Natural Childbirth Institute, pregnant women are advised to stay away from all drugs, including alcohol and tobacco. They are expected to give up caffeine in colas, chocolates, coffee, and tea. Even an occasional glass of wine or cigarette is discouraged. Nancy McNeese said no one knows just how much it takes to make a difference in a pregnancy.

Nancy finds that when she asks during the thirty-sixth-week planning conference what parents want the experience to include, many say, "We want everything the birth center offers." Nancy tells them that the center offers choices and with these choices comes responsibility. There is no right or wrong way to bring a baby into the world. Within bounds of safety, parents may choose whatever seems right to them.

CONNIE, TED AND THE BATHTUB BABY

Even before Connie became pregnant with her second child, The Women's Center of Martin County caught her interest. Her first child, Colin, was born in a large hospital, where she felt like an assemblyline product—just one more passing through. She couldn't wait to return home. Her husband Ted was also bothered that much of hospital procedure—electronic fetal monitor, episiotomy, the cold delivery room—seemed unnecessary. They both resented the defensive measures and shadow cast by malpractice fears.

When Connie saw a news story about a new birth center thirty minutes from their home, she knew that if she had another baby, it would be there. Two years later, she was pregnant and at the center's orientation with her husband. Right away they loved it. Its philosophy of safe, natural, family-centered birth was right in line with their own.

The Women's Center is an airy, relaxing place, with natural wood and bright decor, comfortable waitrooms, and examining rooms. Nurse-midwives provide most of the care. In the Birth House, three homey bedrooms have double beds and private baths. Each bedroom is different, with a common touch: a lace-covered bassinet decorated by an appreciative mother. Families are encouraged to make themselves at home in the Birth House while they wait for and then celebrate the birth of their baby. The kitchen has seen three generations of women bake cookies together—a woman in labor, her mother, and grandmother—while awaiting the fourth generation. The living room, with high cathedral ceiling, opens to a sundeck. A den has a television and day-bed. The center is a cozy and joyful place, a far cry from the strict, impersonal hospital where Connie had her first baby. From the first exam at the center, everything felt so different there. She felt that the people caring for her were her friends, people who were going to work *with* her.

Connie's pregnancy progressed normally. Week 40 passed with no signs of labor. Then week 41. After 42 weeks women cannot give birth at the center; they are referred to the hospital next-door because the placenta could be deteriorated so late in pregnancy, making labor difficult for the baby to tolerate. Connie very much wanted to have her baby at the center and tried to prompt labor with home remedies the nurse-midwives suggested: spicy foods, walks, and finally, castor oil, of which four ounces late one afternoon was just enough to trigger the uterus to contract. By 7 p.m. she felt the first labor pains. An hour later, contractions were coming every five minutes. Ted packed the cooler: lentil soup, Popsicles, apple juice, milk, Cheerios, bananas, bread, and butter. At 9:45, they took three-year-old Colin to stay with a neighbor as planned and drove to the birth center.

The nurse-midwife greeted Connie and Ted. They were the only laboring couple in the Birth House that night. Connie chose the green room—country decor, with a pine headboard and matching chairs and nightstand. They unpacked their food and clothes, and the nurse arrived. They all watched the 11 p.m. news in the den. The midwife listened to the baby's heartbeat, and Connie changed into a robe. She walked around the house, sat, and walked again. She drank some juice.

As contractions grew more intense, Connie stayed in the bedroom, alternating between bed and chair. Then she felt like pushing. Everything seemed right on course, and the nurse-midwife guided her to the bed. To everyone's surprise, though, Connie was dilated only five centimeters. She was so disappointed; she dreaded hours more of labor, or worse, that she might have to go to the hospital for help.

The midwife allowed no time for lament—she got

Connie on her feet and walking, using a table or couch for support during contractions. Then she suggested the tub. In the water, Connie felt weightless. It felt so good that, for the first time in hours, she relaxed. Ted squatted alongside holding her hand, while the midwife perched on the toilet seat. They chatted for about ten minutes.

Suddenly Connie cried out. It felt as though the baby had shot down the birth canal and was ready to be born. Afraid to move, she looked right past Ted, and locked her gaze on the nurse-midwife who held on to her as another strong contraction came and then reached down for a quick vaginal check. Connie was right, the baby was coming, but the midwife asked Connie not to push just yet and opened the drain to draw the water out, while she and Ted supported Connie.

"Go ahead and push when you feel the urge," the nurse-midwife said. "This baby is ready to be born." As the last of the water gurgled down the drain, Sara appeared. With just two or three pushes, her head and shoulders were born. A full forty-two weeks in the womb and her mother's healthy diet made for one plump baby—her backside got stuck! With a little help from the midwife, the 9-pound, 7-ounce girl was soon in the arms of her delighted mother. Connie delivered the placenta, then mother and baby moved to the bed.

The birth was an unconventional one, but Connie was immensely pleased. She relished the closeness and respect she felt in the birth center and the loving support from skilled people who cared about her. Although the delivery was very swift and Sara a full pound heavier than her first baby, Connie gave birth without so much as a small tear.

Ted thought later of the contrast between the births. At the hospital, he waited anxiously through long hours until he could visit Connie and their son, then was told by a nurse not to lie on the bed with Connie. This time, just two hours after the birth, he was under the covers with his arms around his sleeping wife and their newborn daughter.

When they left a few hours later, Ted loved seeing the IT'S A GIRL sign outside the birth center. Sara's name, birth date, and weight were already on the wall that chronicled every baby born there.

"This is a child you are bringing into the world," Ted said. "The birthing center understands this."

TRANSFERS DURING LABOR

Of every ten women who arrive at a birth center in labor, one or two are eventually referred to a hospital. Nearly all such transfers during labor, however, are non-emergency. The most common reason for transfer to a hospital is slow or stalled labor, most frequently with first-time mothers. Standards for transferring a slow-to-labor woman vary from one center to the next. Some require transfer after two hours of pushing or if a woman seems stalled at five centimeters. Others have a woman go to a hospital if many hours have passed, with no signs of labor, after the bag of waters has broken. Other common reasons for non-emergency transfer are irregular fetal heart beat or meconium in the amniotic fluid—possible signs of fetal distress.

A transfer does not automatically mean cesarean. At the Culver City birth center, for instance, 11 percent of all women transfer during labor, but only 6 percent have cesareans. At the Women's Center of Martin County, Florida, the 1990 transfer rate among 272 women was about 14 percent, with a cesarean rate of 5.5 percent. At the Bethesda Center, the 1990 transfer rate was 11 percent of women in labor, with a 3.8 percent cesarean rate. About

DOUBTING PARENTS

The decision to have your baby in a birth center may be difficult for some parents. Out-of-hospital birth may be viewed warily by family and friends who know only hospital birth. But it is your baby and your experience, not theirs.

When Brenda called her mother in New York and told her of plans to have her baby in a Los Angeles birth center, her mother's first thought was "Oh, boy, is this one of those California deals?" Then she reminded herself that Brenda was a sensible person who investigated things carefully. As she heard more about the center, she felt better. From what the grandmother-to-be remembered of childbirth, the center's emphasis on relaxation sounded like a good approach to labor. In a way, she was glad that options were fewer when she had her babies; there were fewer decisions. Despite her trepidations, grandmother-to-be decided not to interfere with her daughter's plans.

"It's her life and her decision," she said. "If I were her age, I probably would be as interested as she."

Some well-meaning friends and relatives may cast doubt on that decision. For the past fifty years, we have been taught that hospital birth with a doctor is the safest option, despite the superior safety records of countries where women give birth with midwives at home. Even Connie from Florida, who was so pleased with the birth center from the start, had a few qualms about safety. Her parents were more concerned; they did not even want to see the center. But Connie knew that hospital birth did not suit her. Her trust in the nurse-midwives grew along with her belly; by her final month, she had no fears. She felt as though the midwives were her friends. She trusted them; she knew they were working *with* her. "I don't think I'd want to have another baby," she said, "if I couldn't have it there."

1 percent of all babies there were transferred after birth; infant transfer is most frequently for observation of respiratory problems. Mothers who transfer after birth, fewer than one percent at the Bethesda center, usually do so for retained placenta or excessive bleeding.

Emergencies, though rare, do occur in childbirth regardless of where mothers plan to give birth. If the umbilical cord precedes the baby (known as cord prolapse), or the placenta detaches from the uterine wall (placental abruption), immediate hospital attention is required. Either of these situations occurs in fewer than one in a hundred births, and most often occur before the woman arrives at the birth center or hospital.

THE NATIONAL BIRTH CENTER STUDY

At least a dozen studies of birth centers were published during the 1970s and 1980s, which pointed to their good results. But one study published in the *New England Journal of Medicine* in 1989 is the most conclusive because of its size and research method.[1] It was designed to address statements by the federal government's Institute of Medicine, which had found that birth settings had not been adequately studied. The National Birth Center Study, as it is known, details the births of 11,814 women admitted in labor to 84 free-standing birth centers in the U.S. Nurse-midwives provided care for 79 percent of the labors and 81 percent of the births. The remaining care was by physicians, registered nurses, and non-nurse midwives. The study excluded women who began prenatal care at the birth centers but were referred elsewhere prior to labor.

Of the 11,814 women who began their labors at the centers 20 percent were transferred to hospitals. Only 4 percent of the total, however, were considered emergencies. Non-emergency transfers were for such reasons as failure to progress, meconium in the amniotic fluid, and fetal distress. Among first-time mothers, transfers were more frequent: 29 percent of the women, as compared to only 7 percent of women who had given birth before. The cesarean rate for women who began labor in a birth center was 4 percent, compared to a national rate of 25 percent.

In all, emergency complications—mostly thick meconium or sustained fetal distress—arose in 8 percent of the women or infants, but fewer than half of these transferred to hospitals, often because the crisis passed and the infant was born. There were no maternal deaths. The death rate of babies from birth to age 28 days was 1.3 per 1,000 births.[2] This rate is similar to that reported in large studies of low-risk hospital births. The rate of low Apgar scores was also similar to studies of in-hospital low-risk birth.

The study showed that one-third of the women, 34.2 percent, delivered with perineum intact and 17.6 percent had an episiotomy. The remaining 45.7 percent had slight tears or ones that needed a few stitches; another 2.4 percent had more serious tears. Of those who gave birth in the centers, more than 75 percent completed evaluations of their care. Almost every one, 99 percent, said they would recommend the center to friends and 94 percent said they would use the center in another pregnancy. Of those who transferred during labor, slightly more than half completed the evaluation. Of them, 97 percent said they would recommend the birth center to friends and 83 percent said they would return for a subsequent birth.

The authors concluded that birth centers provided a "safe and acceptable alternative to hospital confinement for selected pregnant women, particularly those who have previously had children, and that such care leads to relatively few cesarean sections. . . . Fewer innovations in health service promise lower cost, greater availability, and a high degree of satisfaction with a comparable degree of safety.

The results of this study suggest that modern birth centers can identify women who are at low risk for obstetrical complications and can care for them in a way that
provides these benefits."

IF "SOMETHING GOES WRONG"—
CARLA'S STORY

Carla, a first-time mother, chose the Natural Childbirth
Institute in Culver City, California, because she wanted
to be responsible for the birth "and not have a doctor
orchestrate it for me." She wanted to make the choices.
In the end, she and her husband had tough choices to
make.

A full forty-two weeks into her pregnancy Carla visited a doctor for a non-stress test to assess the baby's health
and the fetal environment. Both were fine, the test showed;
they could stay with their plan to have the baby at the
birth center if labor began soon. That very night, her bag
of waters broke. She and her husband headed for the birth
center where a check showed that the baby's heart rate
was normal. With nary a contraction it was clear the birth
was hours away. Carla and her husband returned home.

Weak contractions began by morning, and Carla kept
in touch with her nurse-midwives by phone. By 7 p.m.
the contractions strengthened, and the couple returned to
the center. As the hours wore on, though, the decision
was made to transfer to the hospital—the labor seemed
stalled. As much as Carla wanted to have her baby at the
center, she knew to trust her nurse-midwife's judgment.
The baby apparently was posterior and just could not get
past the curve in Carla's pelvis. The nurse-midwife phoned
the doctor and drove the family to the hospital. Carla was

not sure which bothered her most: the strong contractions or the disappointment of a likely cesarean.

"It was a relief when the doctor said, 'I think I can get this baby out vaginally,' " Carla remembered. He explained the risks—possibly a broken shoulder for the baby or a broken tailbone for Carla. Carla and her husband chose to try vaginal birth. She received an epidural. The baby had turned in the birth canal, making the birth easier, but suddenly the baby's heart rate plunged. To speed the birth the doctor cut an episiotomy and used forceps. A big, healthy baby girl—without a single bruise! It was not the way Carla expected to give birth, but she had no doubt she made the right choice.

"I'm 100 percent sure I would have had a C-section if the whole labor had been in the hospital," she said. With her late pregnancy and long labor, hospital staff may not have been as patient as the birth center's nurse-midwife and consulting physician. "I think we had a lot better outcome because I spent time at the birth center."

Carla felt the nurse-midwife allowed her to labor without intervention for hours at the birth center because of the mutual trust between them, and the trust between the nurse-midwife and the consulting physician. "She trusted us to let us stay at the birth center, to make our own choices [within bounds of medical safety]," she said. "You have to have that mutual trust when you're not in a hospital, without emergency equipment."

Carla had not wanted a hospital birth, with forceps and episiotomy, but she knew these procedures were used for her only because they were necessary. She looked back on the birth feeling that she had chosen a course that was best for her.

"With birth, there's always going to be this element of mystery. You can't control it and you can't understand it," she said. "The transfer wasn't really a disappointment because we did everything we possibly could. And we know that."

COST

Cost varies from one birth center to the next. Nearly all centers have a single sum for prenatal care, basic lab work, professional fees, and delivery. In the early 1990s, a typical fee was less than $3,000—about half the cost of combined physician care and hospital birth in some communities. That bottom line has stunned parents like Connie and Ted. They found birth center care for normal birth to be far more satisfying and at half the cost of the hospital where they had their first baby.

Each center has its own payment plan and particulars as to what is included. Generally, only services provided in the center are covered by the lump sum. If transfer to hospital during labor is needed, the hospital costs and often also the physician fee may be added bills. Therefore, if you have insurance you should find out in advance (1) whether your plan covers the birth center, and (2) whether it will pay for the hospital and physician if you transfer. If your insurer balks at this new type of care, the center manager will likely work with you to see whether they will reimburse, and for how much, before you enroll. Most insurers reimburse between 80 and 100 percent of the birth center cost. Centers generally accept all types of insurance. Many accept Medicaid and CHAMPUS (Civilian Health and Medical Program of the Uniformed Services).

Although prices and services vary from year to year and center to center, these examples will give you an idea of what to expect.

• The Natural Childbirth Institute in Culver City, California, in 1992 charged $3,090 for prenatal care, routine lab work, labor and delivery, postpartum care, and an educational support group for new mothers who delivered there.

• The Childbearing Center at the Maternity Center Association in New York in 1992 charged $3,350 for prenatal care, routine lab work, labor and delivery, childbirth class, and postpartum home visit. The Center will work out a payment plan, but payment must be completed six weeks before the due date. Families who withdraw from the center prior to labor and delivery receive a partial refund. If insurance benefits are collectible only after the delivery, parents must first pay the center and then be reimbursed. The center is included in some local HMO (Health Maintenance Organization) plans. If a woman or baby transfers to the hospital, the family pays all physician and hospital costs.

• In Bethesda, at The Maternity Center, the 1991 fee was $3,200. This includes a few extra perks: two visits to the center's doctors, the physician's fee for delivery if you are transferred and deliver within forty-eight hours, and postpartum visits for the first year. Payment must be completed by the 32nd week of pregnancy. Privately insured women must pay a $200 deposit and agree to pay whatever insurance does not cover. Women who transfer to a physician during prenatal care pay a per visit rate for care received at the center.

• At the Women's Center of Martin County, the 1991 fee of $2,750 included prenatal care, childbirth classes, labor, and delivery. A nonrefundable $350 is required at the first visit to pay for that exam and lab work. The fee is adjusted for women who transfer to the birth center late in pregnancy, depending on how much care they received elsewhere. Self-paying woman must pay by the

34th week; insured women determine how much their insurance company will pay, and pay the balance by the 34th week. If a woman transfers to the center's physician after 37 weeks and has a normal vaginal delivery, the physician's bill is covered by the center.

SHOPPING FOR YOUR CARE

To find a birth center in your community write the National Association of Childbearing Centers (NACC), 3123 Gottschall Road, Perkiomenville, Pennsylvania 18074. Include $1 for brochures, which will be mailed to you. Or contact the American College of Nurse-Midwives chairperson for your local area or state (see page 110). You also may find listings in the phone book under birth center or birthing center, in women's health guides for your community, or at the state agency that regulates birth centers.

Shopping involves asking whether a particular birth center, or any center, is right for you. A birth center is essentially a private practice or clinic and a birth facility in one. Shop as you would for both a caregiver and a birth site. First, list the questions to ask a birth center before you sign up. The answers will tell you what to expect of the center, how it works, and what services it offers. This chapter probably has given you ideas for many more specific questions. Take the questions with you to an orientation, and jot down the answers. Second, list questions to ask yourself as you decide whether a center is right for you.

QUESTIONS TO ASK AT A BIRTH CENTER

Who will care for me during pregnancy and labor?

The answer is probably a combination of nurse-midwife, nurse, and physician. Find out whether you will see the same caregiver throughout and who will be with you for labor and birth.

During pregnancy, what conditions would lead to my transfer?

Be aware of these guidelines, and of the frequency of transfer, so that you will have realistic expectations for completing your prenatal care at the center. Ask whether the center refers women to a particular consulting physician, or whether you would select your own. What is the financial arrangement if you transfer prior to labor?

During labor, what conditions would lead to my transfer?

The answer will give you a better idea of what to expect, and a realistic picture of what the birth center is and is not. Ask who pays the hospital and physician charges if you transfer, and how much they might be.

What are your arrangements, with hospital and doctor, for transfer during labor?

Find out what type of arrangement the center has with its consulting physician and hospital. If a center is not licensed or accredited, there is no guarantee that these arrangements are in place. Think twice about that center. Licensed or accredited centers should have working relationships with both hospital and doctor so that there will be no delay at a crucial time.

How long does it take to get to the hospital? How quickly could you be on an operating table from the time an emergency is identified at the birth center? The answer should be no more than thirty-five minutes, including travel time. Find out what arrangement and rapport the center has with an ambulance or other emergency transport system.

Most centers answer all questions during the free orientations conducted regularly for interested parents. No one likes to think or talk about possible complications, but you must know these answers. Do not regard such questions as impolite or pessimistic. If a center cannot answer these questions directly, consider seeking other care. You need to know that the center has a good working relationship with a doctor, and that a hospital willingly accepts the center's patients.

If I transfer, does the nurse-midwife continue with me?

Nurse-midwives who work at birth centers usually do not have privileges to admit or treat women at a hospital. Some hospitals allow the nurse-midwife to stay with you as a companion. Women find this familiar presence enormously comforting. Other hospitals allow the nurse-midwife to help you settle into the hospital, but she cannot stay.

What safety equipment do you have at the center? Do you use pain medication? Anesthesia? Fetal monitor?

Birth centers do not use anesthesia other than an injection to numb the perineum to repair tears or episiotomies. Electronic fetal monitoring is not necessary for low-risk labor and birth. As you have read, the use of analgesic pain medication varies widely. The answers to these questions will give you a clear idea of what situations a birth center is equipped to handle and what is available to mother and child.

*Does this state license birth centers? Is this center li-
censed? Is it accredited by the Commission for the Accreditation of Freestanding Birth Centers?*

If you are in a state that licenses birth centers, and the
center is not licensed, ask why. Accreditation is a com-
prehensive and rigorous process and has been available
only since the late 1980s. If the center is not accredited,
ask if it has applied.

Will insurance pay?

Almost all companies pay for birth centers, including
Medicaid and CHAMPUS. Some pay 100 percent, instead of the 80 percent coverage for hospital birth. Check
your benefits through your employer. The staff at the
center will help you obtain payment information.

*What are the center's statistics for transfer before labor
and during labor? For mortality? Cesareans? Episiotomies? What percentage of transfers are emergencies?*

A good birth center keeps such statistics and will not
hesitate to provide them. Remember, a high rate of transfer does not necessarily mean a bad birth center, only a
conservative one. Again, some of these questions are uncomfortable to ask, but you should. The answers will not
reveal whether a center meets a certain standard of quality, but they will tell you what to expect.

How soon can I leave after birth? How long can I stay?

Take this answer seriously—exceptions are rarely made.
In most centers, women must stay a few hours after the
birth, but no longer than twelve hours. Some licenses require a center to inform the state if a mother stays longer
than twenty-four hours.

How much baby care do you provide after birth? Who examines the baby before it goes home? Do I need a pediatrician?

Each center is different, and some leave it up to you whether you want antibiotics applied to the baby's eyes or the baby's heel stuck with a needle for a PKU blood test. Nurse-midwives are qualified to examine the newborn; a few centers offer the service of a pediatrician or pediatric nurse-practitioner before the baby goes home. Most centers suggest you choose a pediatrician and begin well-baby care soon after the birth.

Is the transfer hospital able to handle pediatric emergencies? What if the baby is small?

Babies below a certain birth weight, about five pounds, may be recommended for hospital care, as are babies with complications at birth. When you are asking about the transfer hospital also ask whether the hospital has a neonatal intensive care unit, and if not, where the closest one is.

QUESTIONS TO ASK YOURSELF

Do I qualify medically?

The first priority of all birth centers is the health of mother and child. Birth centers will not take risks by accepting women who are anything but low risk. Be realistic. Do not fool yourself or hide any aspect of your medical history that would prevent you from being accepted.

Could I be comfortable here? Am I comfortable with the nurse-midwives, nurses, and doctors who would be with me at the birth?

If the center makes you more excited about your baby, if you can visualize yourself giving birth there, if you feel confident—these clues will make clear whether you and the center are a good match. Listen to your instincts, even if you cannot put your finger on what it is about a center you do or do not like. Remember how Brenda simply did not like the decor and feel of the first birth center she visited, but loved the second. Because tension impedes labor, it is important for you to feel comfortable.

In such an intimate setting, personal rapport with those caring for you makes a big difference. Nurse-midwives are pros when it comes to establishing trust with mothers and families. But if you and she simply do not click, you may want to look elsewhere.

Am I comfortable with safety/transfer arrangements?

You must be comfortable about giving birth without a doctor or operating room on the premises. The same goes for your partner. No matter how much you like a center, if your partner has qualms, they will add tension to your pregnancy and may make you apprehensive about giving birth there.

Can I accept the responsibility for my choices?

Any birth can bring with it unforeseen complications. As pointed out in Chapter 4, however, when parents experience a complication or even death in a high-tech setting, they can tell themselves that they did everything possible, even though the technology may not have helped or even increased a problem. When you choose an out-of-hospital birth, you must acknowledge that you are making a choice outside the current mainstream. You must feel that you have weighed the risks and benefits and chosen the birth setting that you believe in most. The National Birth Center Study and others provide convincing evidence that birth centers are safe and healthy places to have a baby.

Is someone available to watch your other children at the birth center if you want them there with you, or at home if not? Is someone available to help at home immediately after the birth?

Birth centers require an additional adult besides you and your partner to accompany any other children who will attend the birth. And because you will be going home the day of the birth, you should make sure you have adequate help waiting for you. A very helpful husband may be enough, if you have no other children and he is able to stay home from work. Otherwise, think well in advance of what help you may need. You may be quite tired during those first few days and want to spend much of the time in bed.

What do I need for support—medically and emotionally? Does what is being offered match my needs?

Every woman is different and every birth is different. No one except you can know what is right for you. When choosing your birth site, you must realistically explore your attitudes toward hospitals, medical technology, birth in general, and your birth in particular. For many healthy women anticipating a normal birth, the calm, family focus, and joyful approach of a birth center is just right. But in the eyes of some mothers and nurse-midwives, birth at home—with the privacy, intimacy, and comforts it offers—is the ideal setting.

10.

HOME BIRTH WITH A NURSE-MIDWIFE

*"Friends and family who had babies after me
said, 'I wish I had your courage to have a home
birth.' Other people said, 'You're so brave.' It
has nothing to do with courage. It has to do with
what makes you most comfortable."*
—*LYDIA, A MOTHER*

LYDIA DID NOT initially seek out a home birth. She began
her pregnancy with the doctor in Philadelphia whom she
liked so much as a gynecologist. Toward the end of her
first trimester, though, she felt a conflict. The doctor
seemed to insist on more prenatal testing than she desired
or seemed necessary.

Lydia was confused by this unexpected rift. She phoned
a nurse-midwife who had been recommended by her
family doctor and they talked about Lydia's pregnancy
and the midwife's practice. Immediately, Lydia felt comfortable with her and made an appointment for an office
visit. She understood Lydia's hesitance about testing and

Lydia liked her warmth and her attitude toward child-birth. She also liked that her husband could stay in the room when the nurse-midwife examined her.

Lydia wanted to switch her care to the nurse-midwife, but she did only home births. Lydia felt the birth should take place in a hospital. It was her first baby, and she had no idea what to expect. Besides, she and her husband did not want "the blood and mess" at home. She felt frustrated; just the right combination of care did not seem available. Then she met with the nurse-midwife's consulting physician and came up with a perfect arrangement: Lydia would have prenatal care with the nurse-midwife, and the doctor would handle the birth in the hospital with the nurse-midwife present.

Her due date came and went with no sign of labor. Could her slight unease about going to the hospital be holding her back?, she wondered. As the forty-first week ended, she made a decision: she would have the baby at home. The nurse-midwife quickly told her how to prepare.

Lydia felt the same fear and reservation as any first-time mother. But she felt confident in the midwife and confident in her body—and two hospitals were nearby. She gathered the items on the checklist: juice, pillows, a large plastic sheet, oil for perineal massage, bowl for placenta. She laughed at herself for singeing two sets of towels in the oven before she successfully sterilized the third. She enjoyed the tasks. It felt good to be preparing so actively for her own birth.

She awoke the next morning in labor. Active labor was short—eight hours. She spent most of it walking around the house; she was so full of energy she could hardly stay put. "All this stuff was going on inside me," Lydia said. "I knew I didn't want to be lying down. I couldn't imagine being in bed, having a baby that way."

From the earliest contractions, Lydia was in touch with

her nurse-midwife by phone. The birth assistant arrived first, while Lydia was in early labor. The nurse-midwife arrived about an hour later. She immediately checked Lydia's dilation, her blood pressure, and the baby's heart rate. When a contraction came, Lydia grasped a bureau or her husband. Sometimes she squatted. The midwife checked the baby's heart rate often, usually during a contraction and then afterward, recording information about Lydia's blood pressure, the baby's heart rate and length of contractions in her log. She suggested different positions for Lydia to try, including a shower to relax her and later a rest after so much walking around the house. At one point, she suggested Lydia lie on her side, and she arranged the bed pillows to make her most comfortable. Lydia welcomed the suggestions; she liked the way the midwife worked with her, while repeatedly checking her and the baby and assuring her that all was normal. At nine centimeters dilation, the nurse-midwife broke the bag of waters, with Lydia's agreement. Then she suggested Lydia squat over the toilet, which helped position the baby for birth.

When Lydia soon felt the urge to push, she perched at the edge of her low platform bed. Between contractions she rested, sitting on the bed. The midwife continued to monitor her and the baby. When a contraction came, Lydia put her feet on the ground, and squatted, bracing her arms on the mattress behind her. That was most comfortable, and how she gave birth to Seth.

In her own home, Lydia felt comfortable and in control. She thinks that helped her cope with labor and contributed to a relatively easy birth with no complications. "When you are in your own home you don't have to do anything someone else wants you to do," she said. "There's a psychological edge that it's *your* home. It's *your* baby."

Lydia felt that having the baby at home was one of the best decisions she ever made. It also was perhaps her first decision based solely on her own instincts, instead of pleasing someone else. That turned out to be a great way to begin motherhood. At age twenty-five, Lydia was the first of her friends and family to have a baby. She worried that she was too inexperienced in life to be a good mother, but making her own choices about the birth, and being peacefully at home with her newborn, filled her with confidence.

"For labor and delivery to work as well as it can, you have to be comfortable," she said. "I am most comfortable in my own home."

NURSE-MIDWIVES AND HOME BIRTH

Of all births with nurse-midwives in the U.S., about three of every hundred take place at home. Home birth was standard for the first U.S. nurse-midwives in rural Kentucky in the 1920s and 1930s. As birth for women of all social classes moved into hospitals, home birth virtually ceased. Since the early 1970s, however, the desire of women to have more control over their births has brought on a resurgence.

The American College of Nurse-Midwives has acknowledged the safety of home births throughout it history, although training sites for nurse-midwives interested in home birth have not always been available. Some nurse-midwives always felt women were entitled to have their babies at home with professional guidance, and they made the option available. Gradually, more nurse-midwives, and doctors, have become comfortable with the safety of *planned* home birth. Some birth centers include home birth with a nurse-midwife as one of their services. Other nurse-midwives have exclusively home birth practices; yet others offer home birth, birth center, and hospital options.

HOME BIRTH BASICS

A planned home birth with a certified nurse-midwife is a good option for some women who live near a hospital and are at low risk of complications. The woman has the comforts and conveniences of home with less medical intervention. When you have your baby at home you never have to pack, dress, travel, or adjust to new surroundings while in labor. You have your own food, bathroom, and favorite distractions. You have the freedom to define your own experience and surround yourself with only the people you want with you. It also means little disruption for your family and for the baby. To many parents, the only normal way to bring a healthy child into the world is right into the family home. Your baby knows nothing but this warm, cozy, and loving environment.

Nurse-midwives who provide home birth services follow the same standards of care as nurse-midwives in other birth settings. They follow the same prenatal schedule of visits in their offices, yet they usually have more rigorous criteria for accepting women. They may also have higher expectations for you to maintain excellent health and diet throughout pregnancy. Both you and your nurse-midwife must be confident that you have every reason to expect a healthy, normal birth.

As is true for all nurse-midwives, those who attend births at home should have an agreement with a physician who will take on women who deviate from low-risk. Women who become high-risk during pregnancy, thereby disqualifying them from home birth, transfer to the physician for the remaining prenatal care and hospital birth. If you develop a complication during labor the doctor is available to admit you to a hospital and take over the care. Whether you see the physician otherwise depends on state law and the arrangement between your nurse-midwife and her consulting physician. Some doctors see

HOME BIRTH AND NON-NURSE MIDWIVES

When considering home birth, it is easy to confuse nurse-midwives with other midwives, known as lay midwives, licensed midwives, or simply midwives, who also provide prenatal care and assist at home births. These midwives generally do not have nursing degrees, and they have not been educated in a program accredited by the American College of Nurse-Midwives. Many non-nurse midwives have completed a midwifery training program or apprenticeship, but there is no uniform national standard for education and practice of non-nurse midwives in the U.S. Their popularity and practice vary from one state to the next. Some states license these midwives, in a category separate from nurse-midwives. In other states their practice is outright illegal and they work "underground."

Non-nurse midwives may be licensed by your state, have attended a training program, and assisted at hundreds of births, but the level of education requirements and professional oversight varies from one state to the next.

State law, local supply and demand, and the attitudes of local doctors shape the practices of nurse-midwives and non-nurse midwives in each community. In some communities, there are no nurse-midwives who attend home births because none live there or because no physician will agree to consult. Yet non-nurse midwives may be working there. There are ongoing discussions to bring together nurse-midwives and other types of midwives under one professional standard of midwifery.

If you are considering home birth, and want to be sure you are using a certified nurse-midwife, ask whether she is a registered nurse *and* certified by the American College of Nurse-Midwives. The Appendix shows where you can check a nurse-midwife's status in your state.

you once or twice during pregnancy; others see you only if there is a complication.

Nearly all nurse-midwives work with a birth assistant, who may be a registered nurse, a non-nurse midwife, or a woman trained specifically to assist at birth. The birth assistant helps monitor your labor and provides an extra pair of hands at the birth. Most nurse-midwives include the birth assistant's services in their overall package; a few ask you to arrange for your own birth assistant from a list they have approved.

With all the advantages of home birth comes responsibility. You must prepare and clean your home, help the nurse-midwife clean up after the birth and are then on your own with a baby that is just a few hours old. If you are a healthy person and no complications have been noted, the odds are enormously in your favor for a healthy birth. But you must understand the responsibilities and risks along with the benefits. It is a demanding choice.

HOME BIRTH CRITERIA

Nurse-midwives screen women for home birth, and are guided by nurse-midwife standards to accept only those at low risk. Criteria are similar to those of birth centers. Women are excluded for chronic health problems, smoking, and drug use. They must switch to hospital birth if they develop pregnancy-related diabetes, hypertension, or any other condition that would make the woman at risk in the home setting. Some nurse-midwives set geographic limits: no more than a thirty-minute drive from a hospital that can handle an obstetric emergency. Living too far from the nurse-midwife may be another, less crucial factor.

Other criteria vary from one practice to the next. Some have age limits, others do not. A rare few exclude first-time mothers. Because nurse-midwives must know that women who plan to give birth at home are acting responsibly, they may refuse a woman who does not keep appointments or shows emotional instability. A few nurse-midwives allow vaginal birth after cesarean (VBAC) at home; many more believe VBACs can be safe at home, but do not accept women for VBACs because consulting physicians or hospitals object. Some states effectively outlaw home birth by requiring any delivery performed by a nurse-midwife to take place in a licensed facility. The Appendix shows specific rules for each state. Available options and services vary considerably by state and community.

PRENATAL CARE

Prenatal care is the same as with a nurse-midwife in any other setting. One difference, though, may be that home birth nurse-midwives take even more time than others to emphasize a woman's natural childbearing ability. Having a baby at home requires that extra confidence.

"Our biggest job in terms of having a successful home birth practice—and probably for everyone wherever they deliver—is to teach women to trust birth," said Leslie Stewart, a nurse-midwife with Home Birth Service of Los Angeles. "That's really what it's all about. . . . If you can get women to accept that their bodies work well, and they can just trust and let it happen, then that's what happens most of the time. Most of our clients believe that."

If you develop a prenatal complication, however, you will be referred to a physician and disqualified from home birth. Physicians rarely co-manage a birth at home. If labor comes early—before 37 weeks—the woman is referred to the physician and the birth occurs in the hospital. The same is generally true if the pregnancy extends beyond 42 or 43 weeks.

Nurse-midwives who do home births have high expectations of women who come to them for care. They consider an excellent diet to be crucial. Women are expected to stay fit and prepare both themselves and their homes for the birth. Generally, the women who choose home birth are motivated to take on these responsibilities.

"Often people's perspective on out-of-hospital birth is that it is an irresponsible thing," said Leslie, who worked as an obstetrical nurse, a hospital nurse-midwife, and in a birth center before joining the home birth service. "Yet at least within our type of practice, these are the most responsible people you could find. They interview pediatricians and read every book. They ask every question that they possibly could."

CHOOSING HOME BIRTH

Parents who choose home birth must accept the responsibility of a still unconventional option. Birth at home means going without the reassurance of immediately available high technology. But for healthy low-risk women there is no guarantee of a better outcome in a hospital; interventions there actually may bring on complications. At the hospital more germs may infect you and your baby, and medical intervention may start a domino effect that eventually leads to a cesarean section. Other drawbacks are confinement in a small room, nurses who are strangers, and uneasiness over the alien environment. You must weigh the risks and benefits of home birth and feel comfortable with your choice.

The risks at home include conditions that would require a speedy cesarean section. Two situations, cord prolapse, in which the cord drops into the birth canal before the baby, and detached placenta, can occur quickly. But there are warning signs: a broken bag of waters before the baby is positioned in the birth canal, for instance, is a sign to watch for cord prolapse, and early bleeding may signal a placenta dangerously close to the cervix. If a baby's heartbeat is irregular or slow, transfer to the hospital would be indicated. Nurse-midwives know infant resuscitation techniques; but it is preferable, if the need can be anticipated, to be in a hospital.

"You're not going from risk-free situation in a hospital to a risky one at home," said Marianne, a physician in Philadelphia who had two of her three babies at home with a nurse-midwife—the last at age forty-four.

Ellen, another physician (a kidney specialist), also gave birth at home with the same nurse-midwife. She knew long before she first got pregnant that she wanted a home birth.

"I believed what I read and heard about infection rates [in a hospital]," she said. "Infection rates are higher in a hospital than at home, there's so much more pathological bacteria in a hospital. You balance that against the advantage of technology in an emergency.

"There are one or two things, like a prolapsed cord or hemorrhage, that are kind of scary even in a hospital. But if your blood pressure, contractions, and the baby's heartbeat are monitored at home, problems show up early. There's plenty of time to get to a hospital. Things happen slowly. There's lots of warning. There's no reason to be around the technology unless it's needed."

Ellen felt it was safe to plan for birth at home, even though she lived thirty minutes from the nearest hospital. In many community hospitals, she pointed out, it would take just as much time to get an anesthesiologist to the hospital and prepare the operating room if there were an emergency.

With her first child, Ellen went three weeks past her

due date and had to be induced in a hospital because the uterine environment had begun to deteriorate. Her second child was born at home.

"It's so much more relaxing—you have the things you know and love around you," she said. "The sense of being home was important. It was ridiculous how calm I was."

Ellen gave birth in a downstairs family room warmed by a woodstove. Her son, almost three, woke up in his own bed and came downstairs in time to see the birth. She liked how he could be part of the experience, in a place he felt safe.

After the birth, Ellen ate an egg and toast breakfast cooked by her midwife, and climbed right back upstairs and into bed with her baby.

"Things don't happen so fast in birth. It took a long time for you to get there and it takes a long time for the baby to be born," she said. "Problems develop gradually. . . . A nurse-midwife picks up these things early—maybe earlier than someone else would because they are there. . . . Hospital risks are real, and greater than the chances of an emergency at home. It's not that you're risking your life or your baby's. . . . When you're a relaxed person everything goes better."

SAFETY

The professional standards of a certified nurse-midwife for home birth are no different than if the birth is in a hospital or birth center. She is expected to maintain good written records, make sound decisions, follow safety guidelines, and transfer a woman who deviates from the normal. A home birth nurse-midwife is subject to the same peer review and discipline by the American College of Nurse-Midwives as colleagues in other birth settings.

Few studies have specifically focused on home birth with

nurse-midwives, but data are accumulating to show that for low-risk women with good prenatal care, supervised home birth with a skilled attendant leads to outcomes as good as in hospital birth with less medical intervention. Many studies include all home births in a certain area, regardless of who assisted and whether the births were intended for home. Studies from North Carolina and Kentucky showed that the overall death rate for infants born at home was high, but when researchers considered only those births that were *planned* to take place at home, the mortality rate was no different than for hospital births.[1]

Another study, published in 1987 in the *American Journal of Public Health,* found that the death rate for 4,054 Missouri home births from 1978 through 1984 was higher than would be expected for physician-attended hospital births. But nearly all of the excess deaths were with the least educated birth attendants. Births attended by physicians, nurse-midwives, or midwives recognized by the Missouri Midwife Association, showed no more deaths than would be expected with hospital births.[2]

A more recent study published in 1991 in the *Journal of Nurse-Midwifery* focused solely on home births with nurse-midwives among 108 women in two Texas practices. In their third trimester, all 108 women planned to have their babies at home. Of them, 98 actually gave birth at home. Three were transferred to a physician prior to labor: one with gestational diabetes, one with fetal demise at thirty-five weeks in a hospital, and one at the woman's request. Three were transferred during labor for failure to progress. (The remaining three were listed as "missing" and one as "other"). Of the 103 newborns recorded in the study, only four had complications—two had jaundice and two had bruises on their heads. There was not a single case of respiratory distress, hypoglycemia, infection, transfer to intensive care, or neonatal death.[3]

Another report in the *Journal of Nurse-Midwifery* in 1991

summarized all studies of out-of-hospital birth. The authors found that women who plan births at home tend to be older mothers, well-educated, married, white, and who receive early and regular prenatal care. Those who had prenatal care, were low-risk, and gave birth at home with an experienced caregiver had babies that were just as healthy as hospital-born babies. Outside the hospital, costs were consistently lower and obstetric procedures used less frequently. The authors concluded, however, that more study was needed to assess the risk of fetal death during childbirth, although the difference according to birth site was extremely small.[4]

Certified nurse-midwives are taught not to compromise safety to fulfill your wish of a home birth. If there are signs of complications, they will have you transferred to a hospital.

BABY MAKES SIX

"I can't tell you how wonderful it is," said Louise, cradling ten-week-old Oliver. He was her fourth child, but the first to be born at home. When Louise became pregnant soon after moving to southern California, she found a nurse-midwife practice that did home births. She knew the ropes of pregnancy, and was confident after three births in a Denver birth center. She was familiar with the rhythms of her own labor and knew when in labor to call the nurse-midwives. She also lived only ten minutes from the hospital.

Her husband found his colleagues at work surprised.

" 'Isn't that dangerous?' they'd say. But I really don't think so," he said. "You go through a couple of births and you realize, as long as the woman is comfortable, that's what's important. I was very comfortable because Louise was comfortable. She didn't want to have to get everyone together, go to the hospital, come back from the hospital. This was so much better."

Craig and the three children were at home when the nurse-midwife arrived, well into Louise's labor. Zachary, 7, took stock of the birth room and resumed his place in front of the television. Benjamin, 5, lingered at the door, Jillian, age 2½, stayed close to her mother, asking "Is my baby coming out?"

Craig liked the relative calm, and the way the birth was such a natural part of his family's life.

"The midwife hangs out, drinks coffee, talks to the kids. No one gets real crazy," Craig said. "She is right there to say, 'Yup, she's dilated eight centimeters and things are going well,' or 'She's only dilated three, this is going slowly.' "

When the baby crowned, the whole family crowded into the birth room.

"That was so much fun," Craig said. "All the kids were there. Except Ben. He didn't really want to watch the birth, but he came in later when Oliver was all dressed."

Louise had been uncertain about having little Jillian at the birth, and she made sure someone was available to watch her. But the toddler fit easily into the birth scene. She surprised even her mother when she showed how much she understood from the videos and books the nurse-midwives had loaned them. "That's my baby's house," she explained when the placenta was delivered.

Louise loved being home for the birth. Family life could continue without disruption. The children knew just where their mother was, and they knew what was going on. Louise felt being home was the healthiest way for both her and the baby.

"I lay in my bed for ten days with my baby next to me. I nursed him," she said. "He didn't have to be in a cold, bright nursery with a bunch of other screaming babies. I think the baby feels better, I think you feel better."

PREPARING YOUR HOME

When it is time for the birth, the nurse-midwife and birth assistant bring their own equipment, but you are responsible for some other supplies. Early in pregnancy, your nurse-midwife gives you a list of preparations to make and items to have on hand. All must be ready by week thirty-six, including a map to your home.

In a home birth, each nurse-midwife has her own way of doing things. One solo practitioner and her birth assistants, for example, come to your house or apartment for the thirty-seven-week visit, to make sure they know the way and to see that all preparations have been made. Each nurse-midwife makes different requests for supplies to have on hand. This sample list gives you an idea of what you will need.

SAMPLE HOME BIRTH PREPARATION LIST

Supplies

Plastic sheet for bed
Sanitary pads and belt
Large disposable underpads—package of 15
Enema
3 large plastic bags (for trash, laundry, placenta)
Paper towels
Large bowl for placenta; small bowl for possible
  vomiting
Juices or high energy drink, broth
Flexible straws
Crushed ice
Bedside honey jar for quick energy
Sterile gauze pads
Flashlight with new batteries
2-ounce ear syringe

Plastic squirt-top bottle for washing after bathroom use
Thermometer
Two pair towels and washcloths
Four 100-percent cotton washcloths for compresses
Small portable table to lay out supplies
Six large pillows, covered with plastic bags
Heating pad with 4 receiving blankets, baby hat
Ice-filled zip lock baggies
Hand mirror
Olive or mineral oil for perineal massage
Ammonia, to remove blood and meconium
Crockpot to heat compresses
Baby scale (optional)

Other Preparations

—Set up all supplies for the birth and for the baby.
—Place board under mattress if bed not firm; no waterbeds.
—Clean birth room; damp dust daily after week 37.
—Tape together two thick telephone books and cover in plastic, to elevate mother's hips.
—Sterilize towels by warming them in a brown paper bag for one hour at 250 degrees.
—Phone in birth room, with numbers for consulting physician, hospital, ambulance, pediatrician.
—Place infant seat in car.
—Wash baby clothes and receiving blankets, even if new.
—Draw clear maps to two hospitals: the one used by nurse-midwife and the one nearest you.
—Keep car in good working order, with gas tank full.

For Nurse-Midwife

Place to lie down, pillows, blankets, nutritious food and caffeine. Clean hand towel and soap in bathroom.

WHAT THE NURSE-MIDWIFE BRINGS

A nurse-midwife typically brings to a home birth the same instruments she would use in a birth center or hospital: blood pressure cuff, stethoscope, fetoscope, Doppler for listening to fetal heart sounds, baby stethoscope, latex gloves, sterile gauze. A few nurse-midwives carry analgesic pain medication; most do not. Some bring herbs or homeopathic treatments to relax the mother or minimize bruising. A nurse-midwife kit includes episiotomy scissors, suture material, and local anesthetic for suturing; clamps and scissors to cut the cord; vitamin K injection, eye ointment, and sometimes a hanging baby scale.

Most also bring this basic emergency equipment: oxygen tank and mask, for mother or baby; laryngoscope with trachea tube to clear baby's airways; drugs such as pitocin and methergine to control bleeding; intravenous line and fluids.

THE BIRTH ITSELF

When you begin labor, your nurse-midwife is likely to first monitor your progress by phone and may instruct you in final preparations. Nurse-midwives at the Maternity Center in Bethesda suggest you spread the waterproof sheet on the birth bed before labor, in case your water breaks while you are asleep. When labor begins you cover the waterproof sheet with clean sheets. Over that goes another waterproof sheet. On the top layer are clean, old linens you don't mind soiling. After the birth, your partner removes the top cloth and waterproof sheets, and you can climb back into a bed already made, with clean sheets and a waterproof layer beneath.

When birth is in your own home, it is completely up to you who may attend. Some couples want a very intimate birth, with only themselves, their nurse-midwife and her assistant. But if you want to be surrounded by friends and relatives, that is fine, too. There are few rules in home birth, but one nurse-midwife suggests one: anyone who attends must help by bringing food, cleaning up, babysitting, etc.

Throughout early labor you are in frequent phone contact with the nurse-midwife. Because it is essential for you to feel secure and relaxed, she will come whenever you feel you need her or when she feels it is time. As in other birth settings, she tries to keep you as comfortable as possible. She suggests different positions, helps you to the bathroom, and shoos away people if you find them distracting. She monitors your blood pressure, cervical dilation, and the baby's heartbeat. A home birth nurse-midwife may use herbs and homeopathic remedies, and usually uses baths and therapeutic touch to minimize pain and anxiety. She may also use visualization technique, speaking in soothing tones to create a mental picture of your cervix opening wide for the baby. When it is time to push, she helps you position yourself, and works with you and your partner. What is comfortable for you—not what is comfortable for her—is the important thing. It is your birth.

Of the 108 women in the Texas study, just over half had some type of nurse-midwifery intervention during labor. The most common was warm bath or shower (33 percent), followed by breaking the bag of waters after 6-centimeter dilation (18 percent), and stimulating labor with castor oil, cervical stimulation, enema, herbs, or nipple stimulation (13 percent). Although the authors said more study was needed of benefits, risks, and appropriate doses of medicinal herbs, they suggested some home birth approaches might benefit women in all settings. For instance, since women in home births find warm baths and positioning helpful to cope with labor pains, these could be useful alternatives to analgesic medication without the detrimental side effects.[5]

AFTER BIRTH

When the baby arrives, the nurse-midwife examines the newborn, then remains for a couple hours to make sure you are both fine. She must follow state laws for eye drops and other baby care, but there is little other intervention. Some babies born at home seem strangely quiet at first: there is little to cry about in a warm room, filled with familiar, soothing voices, and dimmed lights.

Each nurse-midwife follows her own routine after the birth. As a father reaches to hold his baby, one home birth nurse-midwife suggests he take off his shirt. A bare chest feels nice and warm to a baby, who bonds through sound and scent. As father and baby are getting acquainted, the midwife helps the mother to the shower. She takes advantage of this time alone with the mother to discuss the birth, answer questions, and address any concerns.

A nurse-midwife helps clean up and in most states signs the birth certificate. She helps you begin nursing, then leaves your family napping, taking turns holding the baby, or enjoying a birth celebration. Best of all, you and the baby need not leave your bed, face the outdoor elements or endure a car ride home. You are already there.

Home birth nurse-midwives or their assistants return to your home at least once after the birth. They examine both mother and baby, make sure the cord is clean and check for rash or jaundice. Follow-up visits for mothers are in the nurse-midwife's office at two and six weeks. Moms usually bring the infants, so the midwife can play with the child she helped deliver!

ALI

Ali is a rarity—the second generation of women in her family to choose home birth. Her mother found the hospital so unsettling when she gave birth to Ali's older sister she vowed not to go back. Ali was born at home in 1960 in New Mexico with a midwife, the birth planned that way by her mother.

Nearly thirty years later, Ali became pregnant with her first child. Her friends recommended a home birth service, since giving birth at home seemed so much more relaxing than other options. She knew she would do best in familiar surroundings, with her own bathroom and privacy; her mother's example showed her that home birth was safe. Besides, she was extremely healthy.

"There was nothing high-risk about my situation," she said. "If there were, I'd go right to a hospital."

Her husband's family did not see things the same way.

"They think we're nuts," Ali said. "They have a lot of doctors and nurses in the family. They were afraid. They'd say, 'What if something should happen?' "

Ali's first pregnancy was normal. Jessica, an even nine pounds, was born at home without a hitch. Home birth with a nurse-midwife, Ali found, meant all the comforts of home, plus a birth specialist always by her side to ease the way. Ali especially appreciated the attention after birth.

"It's not like a job where they'll get it done and leave," she said. "They stick around to make sure you and the baby are okay. And they clean up. They know what they're doing and they do it well. My mom started me off on the right foot."

When her second baby was due three years later, Ali and her husband felt Jessica was not old enough to be at the birth. Friends would take the toddler during early labor and return right after the birth. But when labor began Jessica had just gone to bed. Ali decided not to move her. She figured the baby would be born before Jessica awoke.

Toward daylight, as Ali was about to push, Jessica woke up. She wanted to watch. Ali recalled how Jess's tiny, familiar voice helped her focus through the final pushes. Others were probably speaking to her also, but it was her daughter's voice she heard.

"Jess said, 'Look, there's a little nose,' " Ali recalled. "That's how I knew the baby was here."

TRANSFER

No large scale study has been done to provide wide-ranging statistics on the likelihood of transfer in a home birth with a nurse-midwife. Individual practices and smaller studies, however, show that the great majority of women who want to have a baby at home can do so safely. When a problem develops in labor that requires the services of a hospital, the nurse-midwife standard is to call the physician who admits the woman and handles the delivery.

In the Texas study of 108 women who planned to give birth at home, three transferred during the last trimester. Two more transferred during labor.[6] Home Birth Services of Los Angeles, which has delivered more than one thousand babies, has a transfer rate of just over 6 percent prior to labor, and the same during labor. Other, smaller services, report even lower transfer rates. The most frequent reason for transfer during labor is stalled labor, often in first-time mothers. Once in the hospital, the woman may be given Pitocin to spur the labor. For a rare handful of women, the birth picks up naturally in the hospital; some just may not have been comfortable giving birth at home.

Analgesia, episiotomy, and cesarean were all found to be less frequent in home births. Only three women of the

108 in the Texas study had cesareans. Other practices show similar results. For instance, of more than one thousand labors begun with the Home Birth Service of Los Angeles, 2.5 percent were cesarean births.

The relationships between your nurse-midwife, the transfer doctor, and the hospital are crucial. When doctors and nurses see that nurse-midwives use sound judgment, take excellent care of women and babies, stay strictly within the realm of normal birth, and transfer women as soon as complications arise, they become more comfortable about the occasional emergency or stalled labor. Strong backing from the consulting physician and a good track record are important. A supportive consulting physician who is respected by the hospital staff can be a valuable bridge. Few home birth nurse-midwives have privileges to work in the hospital, but many hospitals allow the midwives to remain with women for moral support.

SARAH AND DAVID

Sarah, a sound editor for feature films, and David, a musical-theater writer, fell in love in Los Angeles almost two decades after they had been childhood playmates in Ohio. When pregnancy caught them by surprise, Sarah called Leslie Stewart, who had been her nurse-midwife for gynecological care. The midwife now worked in a home birth practice, however, and that was not how they envisioned having their baby. They simply went to Leslie for advice about birth options.

"We thought, 'Oh yes, let's have a fetal monitor, let's have all this stuff,' " David said. Leslie was the warm, funny, loving, and straightfoward professional Sarah remembered. She told them what happened in most hospital births, what percentage of the time. She explained the options in greater Los Angeles.

"She didn't pressure us at all," David said. "She's not a carnival barker. As she should be, she was very confident. She let us make our own decision."

David and Sarah began to read, and they thought of their friends' birth videos. David tried to put himself in Sarah's shoes.

"I started thinking, 'If I were a woman how would I want to have a baby?' " he said. "Would I want it in a hospital with nurses I'd never met running in and out and a doctor there just for the moment of birth? Or would I want it at home, where everything is familiar?

"We're brainwashed into thinking birth doesn't have to do with the mother, but with how good the doctor is, how good the technology is. But it's the emotions that contribute to a healthy birth."

"Everything we read pointed to home birth," Sarah said. "It took us about fifteen seconds to choose a home birth."

The pregnancy proceded normally. Three days after the due date, on a Sunday, Sarah expelled a clot of blood, the mucus plug, she hoped. Cramps around her groin followed. She thought of calling the midwife to ask, "Are these contractions?" But the twinges came in such regular seven-minute intervals, she figured this was it. When David called to ask if she wanted anything at the grocery store, she remembered the raspberry leaf tea Leslie said was good for labor.

David arrived home at 6:30 p.m. They called Leslie together. She said twenty-second contractions meant the birth was still far off. She would call in a few hours; they could beep her if they needed her sooner.

"You know you are in early labor when you can have contractions and still make dinner," Sarah wrote two weeks later in her journal. "Leslie had said that when I am in active labor I will no longer be comfortable. When it's your first baby, these adjectives don't make much sense.

I was uncomfortable, but I had no idea how uncomfortable I was going to become."

The contractions were the same when Leslie called at 11 p.m. She told David and Sarah to get a good night's sleep. After 1 a.m., the contractions came closer together; they got scared and called Leslie. When she arrived, Sarah was dilated almost two centimeters. She listened to the fetal heart, checked Sarah's blood pressure, and assured them all was well. They probably would have a baby much later that day. She returned home.

Around 5:30 a.m. the contractions grew so strong that Sarah started moaning, which woke David. He timed them: still under forty-five seconds. Leslie returned at 11 a.m.—Sarah was still at two centimeters, so she followed Leslie's suggestion of a warm bath to relax her. She napped, waking with fifty-second contractions every ten minutes.

Then Sarah became nervous. A full day had passed since the first contractions. She wondered how long labor would last. What if it stopped? How much worse would it get? She was not afraid of the pain, but of the unknown. She knew her fear was holding her back.

"It was hard to trust that my body knew what it was doing," she wrote. "Even though I swore I would never consider taking drugs, if I was in a hospital I would have been asking for them. Not so much for the pain, but for the comfort of knowing that in so many minutes I wouldn't feel anything. For this reason I am glad we had a home birth. And there are many more reasons."

Sarah said she would labor on her own; David fell asleep on the couch. Leslie called at 2 a.m. Did they want her to come? Contractions were still more than five minutes apart; Sarah said to wait, but as soon as she hung up, she felt miserable. David could tell she was about to give up. He saw two options: another bath and attempt to sleep, or to ask Leslie to come.

Sarah's gut response was: Now is not the time to sleep.

Now is the time to have this baby. They called Leslie at
2:14 a.m. and gave no explanation for the change of heart.
David simply said, "Come over."

Leslie arrived at 3 a.m., thirty-six hours after labor began. Sarah was propped up by pillows in bed, no longer
smiling or talking.

"Now this looks like a woman in labor," the nurse-
midwife said. She checked the fetal heart rate, took Sarah's blood pressure and performed an internal exam.
Mother and child were doing fine. Sarah was dilated four
centimeters. Leslie brought in two suitcases filled with
her supplies and equipment.

With each contraction, Sarah reached out her arms for
Leslie and David to help her sit. Then she flopped back
onto the pillows. At 6 a.m. Leslie suggested switching
positions or taking a bath. Sarah felt like neither, but knew
Leslie was right. She labored in the warm tub for a half
hour; Leslie held her hand through contractions. She returned to the bedroom and knelt on all fours, as Leslie
again checked the baby's heart rate. The contractions were
closer and stronger. She sensed her bag of waters was
about to break. Leslie put a pad on the floor beneath her;
clear fluid splashed onto it. Sarah felt like pushing.

"The urge to push is not called that for nothing," she
wrote in her journal. "It was something I felt like I *had*
to do." Leslie quickly checked her, found her completely
dilated and told her to follow the urge. Sarah froze with
fear. Again and again, she said, "I'm scared." The mo-
mentum stopped.

Sarah climbed on the bed. She had envisioned herself
pushing the baby out while squatting, but she felt barely
able to move. The first position she fell into, on her side,
was how she remained. Her pushes were half-hearted, but
when she pushed as hard as she could, she panicked that
the baby was not getting enough air. Leslie assured her
otherwise. Marsha, the birth assistant, arrived and urged

Sarah to work *with* the contractions, not resist them. She told her to sit up more, put her chin to her chest and create counter-pressure with her legs. Sarah said she could not move. Marsha said try it once.

"So I sat up and when the next contraction came I pulled my legs up, put my chin down and pushed," Sarah remembered. "I pushed so hard I thought I was going to damage all my organs. And when the contraction was over they said the head was visible.

"Then Marsha said that I might start to feel the ring of fire. Now I'm sure it was mentioned in our childbirth class and I'm sure I read about it in some book. But I had forgotten the 'ring of fire.' Oh my God. When her head crowned I felt like someone was burning a hole in my flesh. Once again I got scared and stopped.

"But then I didn't care how much it hurt. That's when she came. On the next contraction, her body corkscrewed out. Leslie lifted out our baby and put her on my chest."

Sarah heard the words, 'It's a girl.' She felt like laughing and crying, but did neither. She just said "hi!" again and again to little Maddy.

"The next several days we were in heaven," Sarah wrote. "Having a home birth made it heaven. I look back and cannot imagine getting dressed and going to the hospital while in labor. And had I been in a hospital I know they would have tried to speed up my stalled labor with Pitocin. And I might've taken drugs to numb the pain. And who knows, maybe I would've ended up with a C-section.

"Maddy is a wonderful baby and I think it's because we had her at home. She is a relaxed baby who already sleeps five or six hours straight through the night. She nurses frequently and has a smile phase between eating and sleeping. She cries when she is tired, although not when she wets her diaper. She's never been in a nursery with lots of other babies. She's only known what it's like to be in our arms."

DAVID'S VIEW

After reading Sarah's journal account, David offered his view from across the birth bed:

Sarah was a hero. She never became abusive or mean, which would have been more than understandable. When I saw Maddy's hair coming out, I started crying. No matter how much I had reminded Sarah that the baby would soon be in her arms, it was not real for me until that moment. I was trying not to weep, trying to help Sarah, and secretly praying that the baby would be all right—the color of her scalp, etc., was just a dull gray and the more I saw of her head and face, which was gray and lifeless, the more I prayed. Of course I knew everything was all right—Leslie made a comment like "what a cute nose—" so any worries, while real, were more fleeting. What I was really thinking about was that Sarah had no idea how happy she was about to be. I could see the baby, she was a reality for me—for Sarah profound pain was the reality. I watched finally as Leslie corkscrewed Maddy out and she and Marsha seemed to pounce her onto Sarah's stomach. Even though of course we knew what was happening, still, it was somehow a phenomenal shock. I couldn't breathe until I heard that first "Waah!" from Maddy, and then the wellspring of tears really erupted from the deepest place within me. Then Leslie and Marsha said, 'It's a girl!' Sarah was so shocked! I was so thrilled. A little girl! My little Maddy! It was the greatest moment in my life.

SARAH'S DIARY: LETTING GO

This excerpt from Sarah's diary, written two weeks after Maddy's birth, shows how the nurse-midwife was attentive to Sarah's needs, even after the final push:

On Friday, Leslie came over for her last home visit (the next two will be at her office). I cried while she was here and I still cry when I think of her or need to call her. The birth is over. She had told me it might be anticlimactic. I remember when she came in our bedroom on Friday and how the tears just started flowing. I had no idea I was sad. Leslie noticed and hugged me and told me everything I was feeling was completely normal. She also told me that your children grow up and when they're ready to leave, you realize you're ready to let them go. I am not sure what prompted her to say that, but ever since I have thought about childrearing differently: it's about Letting Go. Maddy is only two weeks old, but already she is growing. I remember the first day I put her down in her cradle and how it felt not to hold her. And the night I put her to sleep in our bedroom and then sat with David in the living room. Maddy seems fine, but I cry a little when we make progress. I am just getting her ready for the day when she leaves.

COST

Nurse-midwives generally charge a single sum for prenatal care, home birth, and postpartum care. Most insurance companies reimburse for the services. Coverage amounts vary, but most plans cover 80 percent of the charge; others pay 100 percent. The cost of the home birth package varies from one nurse-midwife practice to the next. At Home Birth Service of Los Angeles the charge was $2,700 in 1992. An extra $100 paid for routine lab work; mothers also were charged for one visit with a consulting physician. In Philadelphia, Lydia's nurse-midwife charges $2,400. Mothers pay another $200 to the physician for two office visits and for his availability during the birth. In some states, Medicaid reimburses for nurse-midwife care at home.

Home birth with a nurse-midwife may be only half the cost of physician birth in a hospital, but if you transfer during labor, you may have to pay the full nurse-midwife fee and the physician fee, plus hospital costs. Each practice handles this differently. Nurse-midwives emphasize that cost should not be the primary basis for your choice. Families that do best are those who feel strongly about having a baby at home, and feel they will be most comfortable there.

ASK YOURSELF

The first list of questions is to ask yourself as you decide whether having a home birth is right for you. The second list is to ask your potential nurse-midwife.

Do you live close enough to a hospital?

Most nurse-midwives follow a thirty-minute rule: you must be within a half-hour drive of a hospital that can handle an obstetrical emergency. Few complications become critical in that time, if identified early.

*Is your home appropriate? Do you feel fully comfortable
having a baby in your home?*

A firm bed, working telephone, and a reasonably clean home are musts. You will need someone to mind your other children. Most of all, you and your partner must be comfortable with home birth and with your nurse-midwife. Just as anxiety impedes labor for some women in a hospital, insecurity about having your baby at home may affect the experience and possibly the outcome. On the other hand, if you love the thought of laboring at home, giving birth where your baby was conceived, and welcoming your child into the family setting, then home birth may be just right for you.

Are you willing to take the responsibility to prepare your home?

Many mothers, like Lydia, find it enjoyable to ready their home for birth. You must be responsible, though, about making the preparations. Your nurse-midwife guides you, but the ultimate responsibility is yours.

Is your partner truly supportive?

More than in any other setting, the role of your birth partner is crucial. You need someone to help you through early labor, to share the responsibility of calling the nurse-midwife, to monitor contractions, and to help make you comfortable. A partner who is just going along may cause you anxiety as the birth approaches. On the other hand, partners who help decide to have a home birth tend to be extremely enthusiastic, reliable, and supportive.

Do you have someone who can help immediately after the birth and during the first few days?

You will be on your own just hours after the birth. You may need someone in addition to your birth partner to free you from household chores to rest. The birth itself creates an extra load or two of laundry right away. Even though having the baby at home helps older siblings feel included, they still may crave a little extra attention.

Are you prepared for the reaction of family, in-laws, and friends who may be skeptical about home birth?

Some couples do not tell their own families that they are having the baby at home until afterward, especially if their parents or siblings may worry or discourage them. Lydia, for instance, told her parents and in-laws after the baby was born. When you tell family and friends, be prepared to explain your choice. And continue to make choices for you, not for them.

ASK THE NURSE-MIDWIFE

The answers to these questions will help you gauge a midwife's experience and what to expect.

Are you a certified nurse-midwife? What are state laws regulating home birth in this state?

Do not make assumptions about credentials. Separate from the practice of nurse-midwifery, some states license non-nurse midwives who do home births. Criteria for licensing vary from one state to another, with a wide range of educational and experience requirements.

How many births have you done? What is your rate of transfer, before and during labor? Have you ever lost a mother or baby? What are common reasons for transfer?

Experience counts. Because you are a step removed from the medical system in a home birth, you want to know your nurse-midwife has handled all eventualities. Ask what she would do if the baby's heart rate dropped, or if you started bleeding. What does she do for shoulder dystocia (when the baby's shoulder seems stuck)? These are not trick questions; they will familiarize you with her approach and with home birth. How your nurse-midwife answers these questions may help you decide how comfortable you are about delivering with her at home.

What conditions in pregnancy require transfer to a physician? What situations in labor require transfer to a hospital? Do you and the physician co-manage women? Do you have a written agreement?

These answers will also clarify what may occur in pregnancy, and will give you an idea whether the nurse-midwife practices within bounds that are comfortable to you. Rarely in home birth does a physician co-manage care with the nurse-midwife. A written agreement also shows a solid relationship that assures you of medical care if needed, although a firm verbal agreement may be adequate.

Does the woman meet the consulting physician?

In some practices they do, in some they do not. Some physicians include an automatic visit or two, to meet the woman and to make their own assessment of the woman's health status.

What is your rapport with the hospital? With the physician?

These are important. You do not want to be transferred to a hospital where nurses and doctors take a scornful view of home birth or your nurse-midwife. Mutual trust between physician and nurse-midwife is equally important. The tenor of these relationships may determine whether the nurse-midwife will be allowed to stay with you if you transfer to a hospital during labor. In some communities, it has been a long, slow road for home birth to win respect. Be aware of this, but do not necessarily let it sway you from the birth that is right for you.

The most important factor when considering home birth is whether you feel truly comfortable with your nurse-midwife. Do you like her? Do you trust her? Do you welcome her in your home? She will be an intimate part of one of the most important experiences of your life. Home birth nurse-midwives tend to inspire enormous trust, openness, and communication in women. These qualities are important as you embark together on the safe birth of your child. Home birth allows great flexibility. Within safe bounds, there is no right or wrong way to have a baby except the way that is right for you.

11.
THE BUSINESS
OF BIRTH:

Cost, Liability and Politics

NURSE-MIDWIVES ARE growing in popularity, not only because they meet the needs of women and families, but also because they are cost efficient. This chapter summarizes issues of cost, insurance reimbursement, and liability for you to consider when choosing your care. It also tells you of the many political battles nurse-midwives have confronted in becoming a part of the U.S. health care system. Although challenges continue in some places, overall the profession is flourishing. In fact, nurse-midwives are becoming so popular that one of the thorniest issues now is how to keep up with the demand for their services as women, health professionals, and government experts recognize the value of their care. The conclusion of this chapter explains how you can play a role in supporting healthy change in the care of women and babies.

COSTS

As we have touched upon, having your baby with a nurse-midwife usually costs less than obstetrical care with a physician in a hospital. The cost of midwifery care usually varies with the setting; most costly is a nurse-midwife in private practice with hospital birth. The least expensive is usually home birth, which may cost a fraction of hospital birth. Birth centers fall somewhere in between. These differences may be significant or minimal, depending on the community.

Having a baby in a hospital involves primarily two charges: the hospital fee and the professional's fee. Doctors and nurse-midwives tend to charge a lump sum for a childbirth package that includes prenatal care, normal hospital delivery, and postpartum follow-up. The hospital bills its services separately. Although charges vary greatly from one community to the next and change quickly over months and years, normal delivery in the early 1990s in a U.S. hospital is on average about $3,000 for the hospital charge and $1,500 or more for the physician's fee. For average fees in your region, contact the Health Insurance Association of America, P.O. Box 41455, Washington, D.C. 20018 (202-223-7780).

In practices where the nurse-midwife is employed by the physician and women receive care from both, there may be one uniform fee. Otherwise, a nurse-midwife's fee tends to be lower than a physician's. Although there is no absolute rule, and variations occur in every community and practice, you'll probably find that obstetricians charge about 30 to 40 percent more than nurse-midwives for professional services. This excludes hospital costs.

When you are in a hospital and receiving care from a nurse-midwife, the hospital bill is generally lower because less intervention is used. The hospital probably charges a baseline fee for the basics of the birth, but ancillary procedures and equipment bring additional charges. Electronic fetal monitor and pain medication each add to the cost; epidural anesthesia alone may cost $1,000. Avoiding these procedures keeps costs down, as does a shorter hospital stay.

When no hospital is involved, costs are considerably less. In home birth, for instance, parents pay only the professional fee, which may range from $2,000 (or less in some rural areas) to just over $3,000. Birth center fees in the early 1990s range about $2,000 to $3,500 for the total package of prenatal through birth and postpartum care. On average, total birth center care in 1989 including laboratory tests, childbirth education, birth, and prenatal and postnatal visits cost less than a single day in a hospital, including practitioners' fees.[1]

When evaluating costs, bear in mind hidden costs that may not be readily apparent. For instance, hospital birth may involve epidural anesthesia, which is not covered by all insurance plans. Or, if you plan an out-of-hospital birth, you may develop complications that require transfer to a doctor before or during labor. Transferring to a doctor during pregnancy could mean you must pay the doctor's full prenatal fee. When you shop for care, ask whether the consulting physician prorates the fee to account for care already received with the nurse-midwife. If you transfer during labor, you may have to pay the full fee for the nurse-midwife or birth center, plus physician and hospital costs. An emergency transfer, while extremely rare, also involves ambulance costs.

In an ideal world, you would choose care based solely on what is best for you, regardless of cost. But the reality is that the high costs of health care play into the decisions of many parents. Diminished insurance coverage is requiring families to become savvy shoppers for health care that meets their needs without emptying their bank accounts. Health-care organizations, as well as individual consumers, are learning that nurse-midwifery care is cost-effective and high-quality. As a result, more hospitals, clinics, HMOs, and doctors are seeking out nurse-mid-wives.

INSURANCE REIMBURSEMENT

Many private health insurance plans reimburse for nurse-midwifery care, regardless of whether the birth occurs in a hospital, birth center, or home. In twenty-six states, as of 1992, insurers are required to reimburse for nurse-mid-wifery care, although not necessarily in all birth settings. Government medical plans, including Medicaid, Medi-care, CHAMPUS, and the Federal Employees Health Benefit Program, all reimburse for nurse-midwifery care. Some insurers have realized that a nurse-midwife birth outside a hospital is less expensive than standard physi-cian-attended birth in a hospital, and these companies provide incentives for beneficiaries to seek less expensive alternatives. At least one insurer reimburses only 80 per-cent of the charge of a hospital birth, for instance, but pays full cost for home birth. Another pays the full cost of a birth center but only 80 percent for a hospital birth.

If you have private insurance, but your state does not require insurers to cover nurse-midwife care or out-of-hospital birth, you may have to pay out of your own pocket to get the care you want. However, do not give up quickly on reimbursement. Call your insurance com-pany and ask whether they cover for the services of Cer-tified Nurse-Midwives. If the person on the line says no, be persistent. Ask to speak to a supervisor—the person on the phone may never have encountered nurse-mid-wifery care. As you explain that nurse-midwives are li-censed in your state, the response may change. You may not always succeed, but it is worth trying. Some families have had claims denied by the insurer, but when the nurse-midwives or families asserted themselves, companies found nurse-midwifery in their protocols. One nurse-midwife said that when a woman's claim was turned down, she sent the insurance company a copy of her license and state statutes governing nurse-midwifery. The insurer reversed its decision and paid for the care.

LIABILITY

Nurse-midwives pay for professional liability insurance, just as doctors, nurses, and other professionals do. That insurance protects them in the event of a lawsuit. Most practicing nurse-midwives are covered by their employers' policies or state-sponsored plans; some nurse-midwives pay for their own coverage. For many, coverage is available through an insurance program sponsored by the American College of Nurse-Midwives. Few states require professional liability coverage, yet most nurse-midwives maintain insurance. If you are concerned, ask your nurse-midwife whether she is covered. Those most likely to be uninsured are nurse-midwives attending home births.

Typical coverage for a nurse-midwife is up to $1 million for each claim made against her, with an aggregate of $3 million yearly. Most policies are on a "claims made" basis, meaning a claim is covered only if the nurse-midwife was insured when the care was given and was still insured when the claim was made. Nurse-midwives pay premiums between $4,000 and $13,500 yearly for that coverage, in a variety of plans. In contrast, average premiums for obstetricians are $23,000 to $26,000; however, in some communities they climb as high as $90,000 yearly. Nurse-midwives' lower cost of liability insurance is one reason their fees remain lower than doctors'.

And one reason nurse-midwives' premiums are comparatively low may be the infrequency of lawsuits. In 1990, a survey on liability issues was sent to 4,000 nurse-mid-wives; 44 percent (1,778 nurse-midwives) responded. Only 158 claims against them from 1972 to 1990 were identi-fied; of these, fewer than 40 resulted in a settlement by their insurance company or a plaintiff's verdict in court. Seven involved home birth. The quality of care or baby's health was not a major factor in many suits; some parents sued because they had not expected to pay the hospital expenses incurred when a hospital transfer was necessary. Some of the other suits involved actions taken allegedly without the informed consent of the woman. Of the nurse-midwives responding, 90.1 percent or 1,602 had no claims against them. In contrast, the American College of Ob-stetricians and Gynecologists has shown that 77.6 percent of their members had been sued once or more.

The initial good health of the women nurse-midwives care for is one reason for the few lawsuits. High quality of care is another. A third, very important reason is the relationship nurse-midwives develop with women. Ex-cellent communication and including parents in decisions lets them know that they are partners with their nurse-midwives for pregnancy and childbirth. Parents who know the factors involved in each decision are less likely to sec-ond-guess, or legally challenge, the decision later.

Women cared for by nurse-midwives also tend to have more realistic expectations of the birth process because they have more knowledge. While nurse-midwives con-vey to families the notion that women and nature are ca-pable of producing healthy babies, they also convey the reality that nature can produce imperfections—not every baby and every birth are perfect.

Professional liability for nurse-midwives has always been a volatile issue. As with most health professionals, insur-ance became harder to find and more expensive in the mid-1980s, curtailing the practices of some nurse-midwives. A June 1987 questionnaire to five hundred members of the American College of Nurse-Midwives showed that higher cost and less coverage led to increases in their charges and in the use of defensive interventions; the changes also reduced job opportunities because nurse-midwives lost insurance coverage, physician support, and hospital privileges.[2]

THE POLITICS OF NURSE-MIDWIFERY

Since the earliest colonial days, nurse-midwives have been agents of change, working to improve the health of women and their babies. In some quarters, however, these relative newcomers have met resistance. In medicine and government, nurse-midwifery has sometimes encountered preconceived, and incorrect, biases about nurse-midwives and the care they offer. Some doctors may have felt their professional role threatened by a new type of caregiver.

Around the turn of the century, as obstetrics emerged as a physician specialty, some states banned midwifery. Midwives of the time were regarded as antiquated and best replaced by formally trained doctors who focused primarily on correcting illnesses that sometimes stemmed from childbearing. As professional nurse-midwifery emerged in recent decades, there have been state-by-state efforts for nurse-midwives to receive legal status and licensing. They have fought for laws requiring that Medicaid and private insurance reimburse for their service, and for laws permitting home birth without accusation that the nurse-midwife is practicing medicine without a license.

Because nurse-midwives choose to work within a framework that includes doctors and hospitals, they rely on support of the physician who is available as a consultant, either within the practice or outside. In communities where nurse-midwifery is new, doctors who affiliate with nurse-midwives may risk ostracism by peers who do not understand the strengths of nurse-midwifery. In some hospitals, nurse-midwives have had to battle with the medical staff before receiving privileges to care for women there. In at least one situation, the U.S. Federal Trade Commission (FTC) concluded that refusing hospital privileges to nurse-midwives would be an illegal restraint of trade. Despite that precedent, many hospitals have no nurse-midwives, in part because of peer pressure among physicians not to provide the necessary consulting services.

Even more touchy is the subject of nurse-midwives admitting their own patients to a hospital. A study published in *Women & Health* in 1989 evaluated the availability of nurse-midwifery services in Washington, D.C., hospitals. The authors found substantial barriers to nurse-midwives; although more nurse-midwives applied for and were granted privileges to work in a growing number of hospitals, only a doctor could sign a woman into a hospital. Physician control of nurse-midwifery was perceived as a major restriction.[3]

Nurse-midwifery is legal in all fifty states, although an uneven patchwork of state laws and local custom influence its practice. Licensing generally falls under the state's Board of Nursing, Board of Medicine, or Department of Public Health. Regulations vary. Some states require nurse-midwives to have written evidence of a collaboration agreement with a physician. Not all states allow nurse-midwives to sign birth certificates. At least thirty-five states and the District of Columbia allow nurse-midwives to write prescriptions for well-woman and childbirth-related needs; the effort to win such authority in other states is ongoing. Meanwhile, states and communities vary widely in the number of nurse-midwives and their scope of practice. In some communities, certified nurse-midwives are still fighting for hospital privileges. Some states have only a handful of nurse-midwives, while in other states nurse-midwives are delivering more than 10 percent of all babies. Other battles being waged are to increase the reimbursement rate from Medicaid, and to receive equal pay for equal work.

One of the most difficult battles, and one that is ongoing, is to require private medical insurance companies to reimburse nurse-midwives directly for their services. In many states, all paperwork for insurance reimbursement must bear a doctor's signature, which restricts nurse-midwives to working only as employees of physicians. It is difficult for nurse-midwives to own their own practices if they are not reimbursed directly by insurers. One of the first successes in winning mandatory insurance reimbursement came in New York, where potential patients of nurse-midwives filed a class-action lawsuit saying insurance companies were discriminating by refusing to reimburse for the type of care women wanted. Gradually more states have required all insurance companies based within their borders to reimburse nurse-midwives directly. This not only encourages a greater variety of nurse-midwife practice arrangements, it also guarantees that more people can choose nurse-midwives without paying significant out-of-pocket expenses.

One emerging political issue for nurse-midwives is the surcharge that some insurance companies, primarily those owned by physicians, tack on to the insurance premiums of doctors who affiliate with nurse-midwives. The rationale for the surcharge is that doctors who work interdependently with nurse-midwives are sued more frequently; but even the American College of Obstetricians and Gynecologists has disputed that notion. The American College of Nurse-Midwives has argued that the surcharge will discourage doctors from affiliating with nurse-

midwives, which could doom nurse-midwifery. It appears to be one more effort to curtail the availability of
nurse-midwifery care.

Another difficult situation has been arranging within
universities for the clinical experience necessary for nurse-
midwife education. Nurse-midwifery education classes
traditionally have been small. Some people say it was to
ensure that only the best would become nurse-midwives;
others say size was constrained by university hospitals that
preferred to fill their limited number of training opportunities with young doctors.

Throughout the controversies, nurse-midwives have
moved forward with confidence and purpose, secure in
the knowledge they were responding to women's needs
in a unique and valuable way. The standards nurse-midwives established for their own education and practice
guaranteed a high quality of care. Their policies for peer
review and discipline added another measure of quality
control and response to public concerns. The results speak
for themselves in the voices of satisfied women.

MEETING THE DEMAND FOR PROFESSIONAL MIDWIVES

The demand for nurse-midwives has begun to outstrip
the supply in some places. A report commissioned by the
New York State Department of Health outlined in 1988
a need for between fifty and two-hundred nurse-midwives in New York City public programs alone.[4] Faced
with growing demand, ACNM has sought ways to educate more nurse-midwives. In 1989 a new community-
based program began, enabling those already holding a
bachelor's degree in nursing to fulfill certified nurse-midwife requirements without leaving their home communities. The program has the potential to enormously ex-

pand the number of nurse-midwives. In the early 1990s a number of new nurse-midwifery programs opened in universities around the country, bringing the total to thirty-seven (including two precertification courses for those with prior midwifery education). Also many of the existing programs have expanded their student numbers.

Meanwhile, an effort has begun to draw together nurse-midwives and non-nurse midwives into a single standard of professional midwifery. It is a controversial effort for two groups that have sometimes viewed each other warily. Some non-nurse midwives consider nurse-midwives too closely allied with a medical model of care that uses excessive interventions. Some nurse-midwives have viewed non-nurse midwives as too inadequately educated to detect problems and too reluctant to seek help. Under the auspices of the Carnegie Foundation for the Advancement of Teaching, discussions have begun to see whether there can be established in the U.S. one type of professional midwife, including an educational path that would not require candidates first to have a nursing degree. A single standard of midwifery in the U.S. is far off, if ever to be accomplished, but the effort acknowledges recognition by women and health authorities that healthy, pregnant women and their babies are best served by caring, experienced professionals who can help them through the physical, emotional, and psychosocial demands of childbearing.

WORLDWIDE MIDWIFERY

Around the globe, nearly all countries have midwives. The word "midwife" describes women of varying education and training, but all together they help deliver 80 percent of the world's babies, according to the World Health Organization (WHO). The International Confederation of Midwives is made up of fifty-two member associations, including the United States, Japan, most of Europe, and many African nations. Statistics year after year from the World Health Organization show that infant health is best in countries where midwives provide the majority of care. The U.S. is not in the lead in this area, repeatedly having among the worst rates of infant mortality for an industrialized nation.

"Every country in Europe with perinatal mortality and infant mortality rates lower than the United States uses midwives as the principal and only birth attendant for at least 70 percent of all births," WHO representative Marsden Wagner told the U.S. Commission to Prevent Infant Mortality in 1988. "The United States should spend far less money on interventionist obstetric care and put more resources into building up a large strong midwifery position."[5]

Despite the overall U.S. record, women in the care of nurse-midwives in the U.S. have an infant mortality rate on par with the countries that have the best infant health. The fact that nurse-midwives here see primarily low-risk women contributes to their good outcomes, of course, but the results are so favorable that health officials both here and abroad have taken notice. Some countries have looked to U.S. nurse-midwifery education programs as a model to incorporate into their own midwifery schools. And U.S. birth centers, largely developed and pioneered by nurse-midwives, are being studied and replicated around the world.

GETTING INVOLVED

Having your baby with a nurse-midwife means taking an active role in childbearing. For you, it may mean seeking out an alternative that is not well known among your

friends and family, but one you know is good for you—
and your baby. Or you may find yourself in the care of
a nurse-midwife at your HMO, local clinic, or hospital.
Whatever the setting, having your baby with a nurse-
midwife means taking the very best care of yourself and
your baby throughout pregnancy. It means being treated
with respect for your privacy, your ability to make decisions, and your choices as a parent. In pregnancy, your
nurse-midwife helps you stay physically and emotionally
healthy as you nurture the baby in your womb. She is at
your side, as trusted professional and friend, for labor and
birth. She is there to help you get off to a good start
feeding and caring for your newborn.

Your relationship with your nurse-midwife need not
end with the birth. Most nurse-midwives provide basic
gynecological care throughout a woman's life. Many
women find having a baby with a nurse-midwife helps
make childbirth an empowering experience, as well as a
healthy one. Just as nurse-midwives have been agents of
change in U.S. health care, you can get involved in the
same goals to provide the best care possible for women
and their babies. Tell friends and co-workers about your
experience, and encourage them to seek care that will meet
all their needs. Call the American College of Nurse-Midwives to find the chapter chairperson in your part of the
country; she can tell you ways to get involved in the political issues that will determine the future of nurse-midwifery in your community or state. More than anything
else, nurse-midwives are about women helping women.
You can help share and spread the collective strength, skill,
and wisdom of this profession that celebrates healthy
mothers and babies.

Appendix:
State-by-State Guide

ALABAMA
Regulated by:
  Board of Nursing
  500 Eastern Blvd.
  Montgomery, AL 36112

Written evidence of collaboration agreement required: YES
Prescriptive authority: NO
Does the state mandate private insurance reimbursement of nurse-midwifery services: NO
Medicaid reimbursement status: Regulations in place.
Does the state regulate birth centers: NO
Status of non–nurse midwives: Licensure for those who qualified prior to 1976. No new licenses issued since.
NOTE: All deliveries must be planned to take place in a hospital.

ALASKA
Regulated by:
  Board of Nursing
  Century Plaza
  142 East 3rd Avenue
  Anchorage, AL 99501

Written evidence of collaboration agreement required: NO
Prescriptive authority: YES

Does the state mandate private insurance reimbursement of nurse-midwifery services: YES
Medicaid reimbursement status: Regulations in place.
Does the state regulate birth centers: YES
Status of non-nurse midwives: Licensed

ARIZONA
Regulated by:
Arizona State Board of Nursing
1645 West Jefferson, Suite 254
Phoenix, AZ 85007

Written evidence of collaboration agreement required: NO
Prescriptive authority: YES
Does the state mandate private insurance reimbursement of nurse-midwifery services: YES
Medicaid reimbursement status: YES
Does the state regulate birth centers: YES
Status of non-nurse midwives: Licensed

ARKANSAS
Regulated by:
Arkansas State Board of Nursing
4120 West Markham, Suite 308
Little Rock, AR 72205

Written evidence of collaboration agreement required: YES
Prescriptive authority: NO
Does the state mandate private insurance reimbursement of nurse-midwifery services: NO. But at least 16 major private insurance companies, except Blue Shield, reimburse for nurse-midwifery services.
Medicaid reimbursement status: Regulations in place.
Does the state regulate birth centers: Birth centers governed by regulations for outpatient surgery clinics.
Status of non-nurse midwives: Legal, with state regulations

CALIFORNIA
Regulated by:
   Board of Registered Nursing
   Consumer Affairs Building
   1020 N Street, Room 571
   Sacramento, CA 95814

Written evidence of collaboration agreement required: YES
Prescriptive authority: YES, for family planning and prenatal care.
Does the state mandate private insurance reimbursement of nurse-midwifery services: YES
Medicaid reimbursement status: Regulations in place.
Does the state regulate birth centers: YES
Status of non-nurse midwives: Not licensed; illegal.

COLORADO
Regulated by:
   Colorado Board of Nursing
   1525 Sherman, Room 132
   Denver, CO 80203

Written evidence of collaboration agreement required: NO
Prescriptive authority: NO
Does the state mandate private insurance reimbursement of nurse-midwifery services: YES
Medicaid reimbursement status: Regulations in place.
Does the state regulate birth centers: YES
Status of non-nurse midwives: Not licensed; regarded as practice of medicine without a license.

CONNECTICUT
Regulated by:
   State of Connecticut Department of Human Services
   150 Washington Street
   Hartford, CT 06115

Written evidence of collaboration agreement required: YES
Prescriptive authority: YES
Does the state mandate private insurance reimbursement of nurse-midwifery services: YES

Medicaid reimbursement status: Regulations in place.
Does the state regulate birth centers: NO
Status of non-nurse midwives: Not acknowledged.

DELAWARE
Regulated by:
  State Board of Health
  Jesse C. Cooper Building
  Dover, DE 19901

Written evidence of collaboration agreement required: YES
Prescriptive authority: NO
Does the state mandate private insurance reimbursement of nurse-
  midwifery services: YES
Medicaid reimbursement status: Regulations in place.
Does the state regulate birth centers: YES
Status of non-nurse midwives: Limits non-nurse midwives to
  populations that are medically underserved or have religious
  tenets opposed to medical practices.

DISTRICT OF COLUMBIA
Regulated by:
  Board of Nursing
  614 H Street, NW, Room 936
  Washington, D.C. 20001

Written evidence of collaboration agreement required: NO
Prescriptive authority: YES
Does the state mandate private insurance reimbursement of nurse-
  midwifery services: NO
Medicaid reimbursement status: YES
Does the state regulate birth centers: NO
Status of non-nurse midwives: Not acknowledged.

FLORIDA
Regulated by:
  Florida Board of Nursing
  111 Coastline Drive East
  Suite 504
  Jacksonville, FL 32202

Written evidence of collaboration agreement required: NO. But
  the collaborating physician must notify Medical Board.

Prescriptive authority: YES

Does the state mandate private insurance reimbursement of nurse-midwifery services: YES

Medicaid reimbursement status: Regulations in place. Medicaid also reimburses birth centers.

Does the state regulate birth centers: YES

Status of non-nurse midwives: Legal, with regulation by the state.

GEORGIA

Regulated by:

Georgia Board of Nursing
166 Pryor Street, SW
Atlanta, GA 30303

Written evidence of collaboration agreement required: NO

Prescriptive authority: Limited

Does the state mandate private insurance reimbursement of nurse-midwifery services: NO

Medicaid reimbursement status: Regulations in place.

Does the state regulate birth centers: YES

Status of non-nurse midwives: No new licenses in recent years; some "granny midwives" are still licensed.

HAWAII

Regulated by:

Department of Health/Maternal-Child Health Branch
741 A Sunset Ave.
Honolulu, HI 96816

Written evidence of collaboration agreement required: YES

Prescriptive authority: NO

Does the state mandate private insurance reimbursement of nurse-midwifery services: NO. But Hawaii Medical Services Association voluntarily reimburses 100 percent of nurse-midwife's fee for birth center or hospital birth; some other insurers also reimburse.

Medicaid reimbursement status: Regulations in place.

Does the state regulate birth centers: None in state.

Status of non-nurse midwives: Not licensed.

IDAHO

Regulated by:
  Idaho State Board of Nursing
  700 West State Street
  Boise, ID 83720

Written evidence of collaboration agreement required: YES
Prescriptive authority: YES
Does the state mandate private insurance reimbursement of nurse-
  midwifery services: NO
Medicaid reimbursement status: Regulations in place.
Does the state regulate birth centers: NO
Status of non-nurse midwives: Not licensed.
NOTE: Fewer than five Certified Nurse-Midwives were practicing in Idaho
in early 1992.

ILLINOIS

Regulated by:
  Department of Professional Regulation
  320 W. Washington, 3rd Floor
  Springfield, IL 62786

  State of Illinois Center
  100 W. Randolph, Suite 9-300
  Chicago, IL 60601

Written evidence of collaboration agreement required: NO
Prescriptive authority: Unclear
Does the state mandate private insurance reimbursement of nurse-
  midwifery services: NO, although many insurers re-
  imburse for nurse-midwifery services.
Medicaid reimbursement status: YES, excluding home birth.
Does the state regulate birth centers: NO
Status of non-nurse midwives: No licensing since 1965. Others
  vulnerable to prosecution for "practicing medicine without a
  license."

INDIANA
Regulated by:
Health Professions Service Bureau
964 N. Pennsylvania
Indianapolis, IN 46204

Written evidence of collaboration agreement required: NO
Prescriptive authority: NO
Does the state mandate private insurance reimbursement of nurse-
midwifery services: NO. But several private insurers reim-
burse for nurse-midwifery services.
Medicaid reimbursement status: Unclear.
Does the state regulate birth centers: YES
Status of non-nurse midwives: Not licensed.

IOWA
Regulated by:
Iowa Board of Nursing
1223 East Court Avenue
Des Moines, IA 50319

Written evidence of collaboration agreement required: NO
Prescriptive authority: Legislation passed, but no rules as of 1/
92.
Does the state mandate private insurance reimbursement of nurse-
midwifery services: NO. Some companies voluntarily reim-
burse for nurse-midwifery services.
Medicaid reimbursement status: Regulations in place.
Does the state regulate birth centers: YES
Status of non-nurse midwives: No licensing, not recognized.

KANSAS
Regulated by:
Kansas State Board of Nursing
PO Box 1098
503 Kansas Ave., Suite 330
Topeka, KS 66601

Written evidence of collaboration agreement required: NO
Prescriptive authority: YES

Does the state mandate private insurance reimbursement of nurse-midwifery services: NO
Medicaid reimbursement status: Regulations in place.
Does the state regulate birth centers: YES
Status of non-nurse midwives: No licensing, not recognized.

KENTUCKY
Regulated by:
  Board of Nursing
  4010 Dupont Circle
  Louisville, KY 40207

Written evidence of collaboration agreement required: YES
Prescriptive authority: Permitted, but not recognized by Kentucky Board of Pharmacy.
Does the state mandate private insurance reimbursement of nurse-midwifery services: NO. Some private companies voluntarily reimburse for nurse-midwifery services.
Medicaid reimbursement status: YES, includes birth centers and home birth.
Does the state regulate birth centers: YES
Status of non-nurse midwives: No new licenses since 1975. Illegal.

LOUISIANA
Regulated by:
  Louisiana State Board of Nursing
  Pere Marquette Building
  150 Baronne Street
  New Orleans, LA 70112

Written evidence of collaboration agreement required: NO
Prescriptive authority: NO
Does the state mandate private insurance reimbursement of nurse-midwifery services: NO
Medicaid reimbursement status: Regulations in place.
Does the state regulate birth centers: NO
Status of non-nurse midwives: Licensed.

MAINE
Regulated by:
Maine State Board of Nursing
295 Water St.
Augusta, ME 04330

Written evidence of collaboration agreement required: YES
Prescriptive authority: YES
Does the state mandate private insurance reimbursement of nurse-midwifery services: NO. But many private insurance companies in Maine have chosen to reimburse nurse-midwives.
Medicaid reimbursement status: YES
Does the state regulate birth centers: NO
Status of non-nurse midwives: No licensing, but no legal prohibition.

MARYLAND
Regulated by:
Maryland State Board of Examiners of Nurses
201 West Preston Street
Baltimore, MD 21201

Written evidence of collaboration agreement required: YES
Prescriptive authority: YES, with limitations
Does the state mandate private insurance reimbursement of nurse-midwifery services: YES
Medicaid reimbursement status: YES, but only if consulting physician agrees to accept Medicaid reimbursement as payment in full.
Does the state regulate birth centers: YES
Status of non-nurse midwives: Not licensed, illegal.

MASSACHUSETTS
Regulated by:
Board of Registration in Nursing
Saltonstall Building, Room 150
100 Cambridge St.
Boston, MA 02202

Written evidence of collaboration agreement required: Nurse-midwives are required to have them, although they need not be submitted to the state.

Prescriptive authority: YES
Does the state mandate private insurance reimbursement of nurse-midwifery services: YES
Medicaid reimbursement status: Regulations in place.
Does the state regulate birth centers: YES
Status of non-nurse midwives: No licensing, but not illegal.

MICHIGAN

Regulated by:
Board of Nursing
905 Southland
PO Box 30018
Lansing, MI 48909

Written evidence of collaboration agreement required: NO
Prescriptive authority: YES, if delegated by MD.
Does the state mandate private insurance reimbursement of nurse-midwifery services: NO. But Blue Cross/Blue Shield began covering nurse-midwifery services in 1992.
Medicaid reimbursement status: YES, with physician's written collaboration agreement.
Does the state regulate birth centers: None in state.
Status of non-nurse midwives: No new licenses.

MINNESOTA

Regulated by:
Board of Nursing
Department of Health
717 Delaware Street, SE
Minneapolis, MN 55414

Written evidence of collaboration agreement required: NO
Prescriptive authority: YES
Does the state mandate private insurance reimbursement of nurse-midwifery services: YES
Medicaid reimbursement status: Regulations in place.
Does the state regulate birth centers: NO
Status of non-nurse midwives: No new licenses since 1939.

MISSISSIPPI
Regulated by:
Mississippi Board of Nursing
135 Bounds Street
Jackson, MS 39206

Written evidence of collaboration agreement required: YES
Prescriptive authority: YES
Does the state mandate private insurance reimbursement of nurse-midwifery services: YES. But claim forms must be signed by physician.
Medicaid reimbursement status: Regulations in place.
Does the state regulate birth centers: YES
Status of non-nurse midwives: License not required for the practice of midwifery.

MISSOURI
Regulated by:
Board of Nursing
PO Box 656
3523 North Ten Mile Drive
Jefferson City, MO 65102

Written evidence of collaboration agreement required: NO
Prescriptive authority: NO
Does the state mandate private insurance reimbursement of nurse-midwifery services: NO. Some companies reimburse voluntarily.
Medicaid reimbursement status: Regulations in place.
Does the state regulate birth centers: NO
Status of non-nurse midwives: No new licenses since 1959.

MONTANA
Regulated by:
Board of Nursing
Department of Commerce
1424 Ninth Avenue
Helena, MT 59620

Written evidence of collaboration agreement required: NO.
Nurse-midwives need only show a "means of referral" in

case of emergency, which can include an emergency room in a nearby hospital or a list of physicians available.

Prescriptive authority: YES

Does the state mandate private insurance reimbursement of nurse-midwifery services: YES

Medicaid reimbursement status: Regulations in place.

Does the state regulate birth centers: NO

Status of non-nurse midwives: Work under state license, with education and experience requirements.

NEBRASKA

Regulated by:
  Board of Nursing
  301 Centennial Mall South
  Lincoln, NE 68509

Written evidence of collaboration agreement required: YES

Prescriptive authority: Limited

Does the state mandate private insurance reimbursement of nurse-midwifery services: NO

Medicaid reimbursement status: YES

Does the state regulate birth centers: NO

Status of non-nurse midwives: Not licensed.

NOTES: CNMs may not attend home births. Only one nurse-midwife was practicing in Nebraska in the early 1990s.

NEVADA

Regulated by:
  Nevada Board of Nursing
  1135 Terminal Way, Room 209
  Reno, NV 89502

Written evidence of collaboration agreement required: YES

Prescriptive authority: YES

Does the state mandate private insurance reimbursement of nurse-midwifery services: YES

Medicaid reimbursement status: Unknown

Does the state regulate birth centers: NO

Status of non-nurse midwives: Not licensed.

NEW HAMPSHIRE
Regulated by:
New Hampshire Board of Nursing
Registration and Education
Loudon Road
Concord, NH 03301

Written evidence of collaboration agreement required: YES
Prescriptive authority: YES
Does the state mandate private insurance reimbursement of nurse-
midwifery services: YES
Medicaid reimbursement status: YES
Does the state regulate birth centers: YES, but as of 1992 there
were none.
Status of non-nurse midwives: State certification.

NEW JERSEY
Regulated by:
Department of Law and Public Safety
Division of Consumer Affairs
Board of Medical Examiners
28 West State Street
Trenton, NJ 08608

Written evidence of collaboration agreement required: YES
Prescriptive authority: YES
Does the state mandate private insurance reimbursement of nurse-
midwifery services: YES
Medicaid reimbursement status: YES
Does the state regulate birth centers: YES
Status of non-nurse midwives: Regulated by the state, with
specific rules for practice.

NEW MEXICO
Regulated by:
Department of Health
Maternal and Child Health Bureau
PO Box 26110
Santa Fe, NM 87502

Written evidence of collaboration agreement required: YES
Prescriptive authority: YES
Does the state mandate private insurance reimbursement of nurse-midwifery services: YES
Medicaid reimbursement status: Regulations in place.
Does the state regulate birth centers: YES
Status of non-nurse midwives: Work under state license.

NEW YORK
Regulated by:
New York State Department of Health
Division of Health Manpower
Tower Building
Empire State Plaza
Albany, NY 12237

Written evidence of collaboration agreement required: YES
Prescriptive authority: YES, if also licensed as nurse-practitioner.
Does the state mandate private insurance reimbursement of nurse-midwifery services: YES
Medicaid reimbursement status: Regulations in place.
Does the state regulate birth centers: YES
Status of non-nurse midwives: Illegal.

NORTH CAROLINA
Regulated by:
Midwifery Joint Committee
PO Box 2129
Raleigh, NC 27602

Written evidence of collaboration agreement required: YES
Prescriptive authority: YES
Does the state mandate private insurance reimbursement of nurse-midwifery services: NO

Medicaid reimbursement status: YES
Does the state regulate birth centers: NO
Status of non-nurse midwives: Only those working prior to
   1973 are legal.

NORTH DAKOTA
Regulated by:
   Board of Nursing
   919 S. 7th Street Suite 504
   Bismarck, ND 58504-5881

Written evidence of collaboration agreement required: YES
Prescriptive authority: YES
Does the state mandate private insurance reimbursement of nurse-
   midwifery services: NO
Medicaid reimbursement status: Uncertain.
Does the state regulate birth centers: NO
Status of non-nurse midwives: Not licensed; not recognized.

OHIO
Regulated by:
   Ohio State Medical Board
   65 South Front Street
   Columbus, OH 43215

Written evidence of collaboration agreement required: NO
Prescriptive authority: NO
Does the state mandate private insurance reimbursement of nurse-
   midwifery services: YES
Medicaid reimbursement status: Regulations in place.
Does the state regulate birth centers: NO
Status of non-nurse midwives: No licensing, not recognized.

OKLAHOMA
Regulated by:
   Board of Nursing
   2915 N. Classen Blvd. Suite 524
   Oklahoma City, OK 73106-5437

Written evidence of collaboration agreement required: NO
Prescriptive authority: NO

Does the state mandate private insurance reimbursement of nurse-midwifery services: NO
Medicaid reimbursement status: YES
Does the state regulate birth centers: YES
Status of non-nurse midwives: Not licensed.

OREGON
Regulated by:
Oregon State Board of Nursing
1200 S.W. 5th Avenue
Portland, OR 97201

Written evidence of collaboration agreement required: NO
Prescriptive authority: YES
Does the state mandate private insurance reimbursement of nurse-midwifery services: YES
Medicaid reimbursement status: Regulations in place.
Does the state regulate birth centers: YES
Status of non-nurse midwives: Not licensed, but practice widely and have created a self-governing organization.

PENNSYLVANIA
Regulated by:
Board of Medical Education and Licensure
PO Box 2649
Transportation and Safety Building
Commonwealth and Forster Streets
Harrisburg, PA 17120

Written evidence of collaboration agreement required: YES
Prescriptive authority: NO
Does the state mandate private insurance reimbursement of nurse-midwifery services: YES
Medicaid reimbursement status: Regulations in place.
Does the state regulate birth centers: YES
Status of non-nurse midwives: Illegal

PUERTO RICO
Regulated by:
  State Board of Nurse Examiners
  Departmento de Salud
  Junta Examinadora
  San Juan, PR

Written evidence of collaboration agreement required: NO
Prescriptive authority: NO
Does the state mandate private insurance reimbursement of nurse-midwifery services: NO
Medicaid reimbursement status: Unknown.
Does the state regulate birth centers: NO
Status of non-nurse midwives: No new licenses.

RHODE ISLAND
Regulated by:
  Division of Professional Regulation
  Rhode Island State Health Department
  Davis St.
  Providence, RI 02729

Written evidence of collaboration agreement required: NO
Prescriptive authority: YES
Does the state mandate private insurance reimbursement of nurse-midwifery services: YES
Medicaid reimbursement status: Regulations in place.
Does the state regulate birth centers: NO
Status of non-nurse midwives: State license with education requirements.

SOUTH CAROLINA
Regulated by:
  State Board of Nursing for South Carolina
  220 Executive Drive, Suite 220
  Columbia, SC 29210

Written evidence of collaboration agreement required: Uncertain
Prescriptive authority: Uncertain

Does the state mandate private insurance reimbursement of nurse-midwifery services: NO
Medicaid reimbursement status: YES. For maternity services only.
Does the state regulate birth centers: NO
Status of non-nurse midwives: Licensed.

SOUTH DAKOTA
Regulated by:
South Dakota Board of Nursing
304 South Phillips Avenue Suite 205
Sioux Falls, SD 57102

Written evidence of collaboration agreement required: YES
Prescriptive authority: YES
Does the state mandate private insurance reimbursement of nurse-midwifery services: YES
Medicaid reimbursement status: Unknown
Does the state regulate birth centers: NO
Practice settings restricted to: Public health agency, affiliation with licensed or certified health care agency, office, or supervision of a licensed physician.
Status of non-nurse midwives: No licensing, not recognized.

TENNESSEE
Regulated by:
Tennessee State Board of Nursing
283 Plus Park Boulevard
Nashville, TN 37219-5407

Written evidence of collaboration agreement required: NO
Prescriptive authority: YES
Does the state mandate private insurance reimbursement of nurse-midwifery services: NO
Medicaid reimbursement status: YES
Does the state regulate birth centers: YES
Status of non-nurse midwives: Not regulated, but not illegal.

TEXAS
Regulated by:
Board of Nurse Examiners
1300 E. Anderson Lane
Building C, Suite 225
Austin, TX 78752

Written evidence of collaboration agreement required: YES
Prescriptive authority: YES, as delegated by physician.
Does the state mandate private insurance reimbursement of nurse-midwifery services: NO
Medicaid reimbursement status: YES. Home birth reimbursement requires physician approval.
Does the state regulate birth centers: YES
Status of non-nurse midwives: Regulated by the state.

UTAH
Regulated by:
Division of Occupational and Professional Licensing
Department of Business Regulation
160 East 300 So. Street
PO Box 45802
Salt Lake City, UT 84145-0801

Written evidence of collaboration agreement required: YES
Prescriptive authority: YES
Does the state mandate private insurance reimbursement of nurse-midwifery services: YES
Medicaid reimbursement status: Regulations in place.
Does the state regulate birth centers: YES
Status of non-nurse midwives: Not licensed, but not prohibited.

VERMONT
Regulated by:
  Vermont Board of Nursing
  Pavilion Office Building
  26 Terrace Street
  Montpelier, VT 05602

Written evidence of collaboration agreement required: YES
Prescriptive authority: YES
Does the state mandate private insurance reimbursement of nurse-midwifery services: NO. But most private insurers voluntarily reimburse for nurse-midwifery services.
Medicaid reimbursement status: Regulations in place.
Does the state regulate birth centers: NO
Status of non-nurse midwives: No licensing.

VIRGIN ISLANDS
Regulated by:
  Virgin Islands Board of Nurse Licensure
  PO Box 7309
  St. Thomas, VI 00801

Written evidence of collaboration agreement required: NO
Prescriptive authority: NO
Does the state mandate private insurance reimbursement of nurse-midwifery services: NO
Medicaid reimbursement status: Not applicable.
Does the state regulate birth centers: NO
Status of non-nurse midwives: No legal authorization.

VIRGINIA
Regulated by:
  Department of Health Professions
  Virginia State Board of Nursing
  1601 Rolling Hill Drive, Suite 200
  Richmond, VA 23229-5005

Written evidence of collaboration agreement required: NO
Prescriptive authority: YES
Does the state mandate private insurance reimbursement of nurse-

midwifery services: NO. But most private insurers voluntarily reimburse for nurse-midwifery services.

Medicaid reimbursement status: Regulations in place. Requires physician signature.

Does the state regulate birth centers: NO

Status of non-nurse midwives: No new licenses since 1976.

WASHINGTON

Regulated by:
   State Board of Nursing
   Division of Professional Licensing
   Box 9649
   Olympia, WA 98504

Written evidence of collaboration agreement required: NO

Prescriptive authority: YES

Does the state mandate private insurance reimbursement of nurse-midwifery services: YES

Medicaid reimbursement status: YES

Does the state regulate birth centers: YES

Status of non-nurse midwives: Work under state license, after three years of study and other requirements.

WEST VIRGINIA

Regulated by:
   Board of Examiners for Registered Professional Nurses
   1800 Washington Street East, Room 416
   Charleston, West Virginia 25305

Written evidence of collaboration agreement required: NO

Prescriptive authority: NO

Does the state mandate private insurance reimbursement of nurse-midwifery services: YES

Medicaid reimbursement status: YES

Does the state regulate birth centers: Regulations in place.

Status of non-nurse midwives: Licensing ended with a 1973 law, which permits only nurse-midwives and physicians to practice midwifery.

WISCONSIN
Regulated by:
Department of Regulation and Licensing
Bureau of Nursing
PO Box 8936
Madison, WI 53708

Written evidence of collaboration agreement required: YES
Prescriptive authority: YES
Does the state mandate private insurance reimbursement of nurse-
midwifery services: NO
Medicaid reimbursement status: YES
Does the state regulate birth centers: NO
Status of non–nurse midwives: No licensing; not recognized.

WYOMING
Regulated by:
Wyoming State Board of Nursing
2223 Warren Avenue, Suite One
Cheyenne, WY 82002

Written evidence of collaboration agreement required: YES
Prescriptive authority: YES
Does the state mandate private insurance reimbursement of nurse-
midwifery services: YES
Medicaid reimbursement status: Rules in place.
Does the state regulate birth centers: NO
Status of non–nurse midwives: No licensing.

Sources
Bidgood Wilson, M.; Barickman, C., Ackley, S., Nurse-Mid-
wifery Today, A Legislative Update, Parts I and II. *Journal
of Nurse-Midwifery* 37, (2) (1992):96–140 and 37, (3) (1992):175–
214.
Mothering Special Edition, compiled by Becker, Ellie; Long,
Marie; Stamler, Vicki; Sallomi, Pacia. *Midwifery and the Law.*
Santa Fe: Peggy O'Mara, 1990.

Notes

Chapter One

1. Richard W. and Dorothy C. Wertz, *Lying-In, a History of Childbirth in America* (New York: The Free Press, 1977), 162.
2. Ibid., 164.
3. The National Center for Health Statistics, U.S. Department of Health and Human Services, *Advance Report of Final Natality Statistics, 1989.* Monthly Vital Statistics Report, Vol. 40, No. 8, supplement (December 12, 1991), 25. Of all births attended by nurse-midwives, about 93 percent were in hospitals, 4.5 percent in birth centers and the remaining 2.5 percent in homes, according to figures from the National Center for Health Statistics, U.S. Department of Health and Human Services.
4. Nurse-midwives who attend hospital births generally average more births in a year.

Chapter Two

1. M. Avery, and B. Burket, "Effect of perineal massage on the incidence of episiotomy and perineal laceration in a nurse-midwifery service." *Journal of Nurse-Midwifery,* 31 (3) (1986):128–134.

Chapter Four

1. Sheila Kitzinger, *Your Baby, Your Way.* (New York: Pantheon Books, 1987), 269–270.
2. J. Rooks, N. Weatherby, E. Ernst, S. Stapleton, D. Rosen, A. Rosenfeld, "Outcomes of care in birth centers: The na-

tional birth center study." *New England Journal of Medicine,* 321 (26) (1989):1804–1811. The authors noted, however, that the expected incidence of aspiration under anesthesia— 1 in 2,000—was such that the practice of eating during labor still should be questioned, despite the absence of complications observed in the sample.

3. These studies are noted and summarized in the March 1, 1990, *New England Journal of Medicine,* "The Effects of Electronic Fetal-Heart-Rate Monitoring, as Compared with Periodic Ascultation, on the Neurological Development of Premature Infants," by Kirkwood Shy et al., 588–593, and in the same issue, an editorial "Intrapartum Fetal Monitoring—A Disappointing Story," by Roger Freeman, 624–626.

4. American College of Obstetricians and Gynecologists Technical Bulletin #132, "Intrapartum Fetal Heart Rate Monitoring (September 1989):2.

5. American College of Obstetricians and Gynecologists Committee Opinion Number 64, "Guidelines for Vaginal Delivery After Cesarean Birth" (October 1988).

6. N. Bowe, "Intact perineum: A slow delivery of the head does not adversely affect the outcome of the newborn." *Journal of Nurse-Midwifery,* 26 (2) (1981):5–11.

7. J. Fardig, "Comparison of skin-to-skin contact and radiant heaters in promoting neonatal thermal regulation." *Journal of Nurse-Midwifery,* 25 (1) (1980):19–28.

Chapter Six

1. C. Krutsky, "Sibling at birth: Impact on parents." *Journal of Nurse-Midwifery,* 30 (5) (1985):269–276.

2. G. DelGiudice, "The relationship between sibling jealousy and presence at a sibling's birth." *Birth,* 13 (4) (1986):250–254.

Chapter Seven

1. United States Congress, Office of Technology Assessment. Nurse Practitioners, Physicians Assistants, and Certified Nurse-Midwives: A Policy Analysis (Washington, D.C.: U.S. Government Printing Office, 1986):5–6. [Health Technology Case Study 37]

2. Neonatal death refers to death of an infant within 28 days of birth. M.D. Laird, "Report of the maternity center association clinic, New York 1931—1951. *American Journal of Obstetrics and Gynecology* 69 (1955):178–184.

3. J. Thompson, "Nurse-midwifery care: 1925–1984." *In H.H. Werley, J.J. Fitzpatrick, R.L. Taunton* (eds.), Annual Review of Nursing Research 4 (1986):164. Thompson's summary of FNS is based on three prior studies.

4. B.S. Levy, F.S. Wilkinson, W.M. Marine, "Reducing neonatal mortality rate with nurse-midwives." *American Journal of Obstetrics & Gynecology,* 109 (1971):51–58.

5. C. Slome, M. Wetherbee, M. Daly, K. Christensen, M. Meglen, H. Thiede, Effectiveness of Certified Nurse-Midwives. *American Journal of Obstetrics and Gynecology* 124 (1976):177–182.

6. M. Beale, Nurse-Midwifery intrapartum management. *Journal of Nurse-Midwifery,* 29 (1) (1984):13–19.

7. K. Bell, and J. Mills, "Certified nurse-midwife effectiveness in the health maintenance organization obstetric team." *Obstetrics and Gynecology,* 74 (1) (1989):112–116.

8. G. Baruffi, W. Dellinger, D. Strobino, A. Rudolph, R. Timmons, and A. Ross, "A study of pregnancy outcomes in a maternity center and tertiary care hospital." *American Journal of Public Health* 74 (9) (1984):973–978.

9. D. Strobino, G. Baruffi, W. Dellinger, A. Ross, "Variations in pregnancy outcomes and use of procedures in two institutions with divergent philosophies of maternity care." *Medical Care* 26 (4) (1988):337–347.

10. G. Baruffi, W. Dellinger, D. Strobino, A. Rudolph, R. Timmons, and A. Ross, "Patterns of obstetric procedure used in maternity care." *Obstetrics and Gynecology* 64 (4) (1984):493–498.

11. G. Baruffi, D. Strobino, L. Paine, "Investigation of Institutional Differences in Primary Cesarean Birth Rates." *Journal of Nurse-Midwifery* 35 (5) (1990):274–281.

12. Strobino et al., *Medical Care,* 973–978.

13. Baruffi et al., *Obstetrics and Gynecology,* 493–498.

14. Ibid.

15. Ibid.

16. L. Davis, "The use of castor oil to stimulate labor in patients with premature rupture of membranes." *Journal of Nurse-Midwifery*, 29 (6) (1984):366–370.
17. E. Birch, "The experience of touch received during labor," *Journal of Nurse-Midwifery*, 31 (6) (1986):270–76.
18. B. Bills, "Enhancement of paternal-newborn affectional bonds." *Journal of Nurse-Midwifery* 25 (5) (1980):21–26.
19. K. Norr, J. Roberts, V. Freese, "Early postpartum rooming-in and maternal attachment behaviors in a group of medically indigent primiparas." *Journal of Nurse-Midwifery* 34 (2) (1989):85–91.
20. C. Nichols, "Postdate pregnancy." *Journal of Nurse-Midwifery*, 30 (4) (1985):222–238.
21. M. Poore, and J. Foster, "Epidural and no epidural anesthesia: Differences between mothers and their experience of birth." *Birth* 12 (4) (1985):205–212.
22. K. Stolte, "A comparison of women's expectations of labor with the actual event." *Birth* 14 (2) (1987):99–103.
23. R. Freeman, "Intrapartum fetal monitoring—a disappointing story." *The New England Journal of Medicine*. (March 1, 1990):624–626.
24. N. Bowe, "Intact perineum: A slow delivery of the head does not adversely affect the outcome of the newborn," *Journal of Nurse-Midwifery* 26 (2) (1981):5–11.
25. L. Formato, "Routine Prophylactic Episiotomy," *Journal of Nurse-Midwifery* 30 (3) (1985):144–148.
26. M. McGuinness, K. Norr, K. Nacion, "Comparison Between Different Perineal Outcomes on Tissue Healing," *Journal of Nurse-Midwifery* 36 (3) (1991):192–198.
27. R. Wilf, and J. Franklin, "Six years' experience with vaginal births after cesareans at Booth Maternity Center in Philadelphia," *Birth* 11 (1) (1984):5–9.
28. K. Hangsleben, M. Taylor, and N. Lynn, "VBAC program in a nurse-midwifery service," *Journal of Nurse-Midwifery* 34 (4) (1989):179–184.
29. J. Rooks, N. Weatherby, E. Ernst, S. Stapleton, D. Rosen, A. Rosenfeld, "Outcomes of care in birth centers: The national birth center study." *The New England Journal of Medicine* 321 (26) (1989):1804–1811.

30. S. Piechnik, and M. Corbett, "Reducing low birth weight among socioeconomically high-risk adolescent pregnancies," *The Journal of Nurse-Midwifery* 30 (2) (1985):88–98.

31. M. Brucker, and M. Muellner, "Nurse-Midwifery care of adolescents," *Journal of Nurse-Midwifery* 30 (5) (1985):277–279.

32. National Academy of Sciences, Institute of Medicine, *Preventing Low Birthweight* (Washington, D.C.: National Academy Press, 1985).

33. United States Congress, Office of Technology Assessment, *Nurse-Practitioners, Physicians Assistants, and Certified Nurse-Midwives: A Policy Analysis* (Washington, D.C.: U.S. GPO; 1986).

34. Institute of Medicine, *Prenatal Care: Reaching Mothers, Reaching Infants.* Sarah S. Brown, editor (Washington, D.C.: National Academy Press, 1988).

35. The National Commission to Prevent Infant Mortality, *Death Before Life: The Tragedy of Infant Mortality.* (Washington, D.C., August 1988).

Chapter Nine

1. J. Rooks, N. Weatherby, E. Ernst, S. Stapleton, D. Rosen, A. Rosenfeld, "Outcomes of care in birth centers: The national birth center study." *The New England Journal of Medicine* 321 (26) (1989):1804–1811.

2. Ibid. This is lower than indicated in prior birth center studies. A study of 1938 women in 11 birth centers from 1972 to 1979 showed a neonatal mortality rate of 4.6 per 1,000 births. There were 4 neonatal deaths per 1,000 births among 2,002 admissions to 16 California birth centers in 1984. An assessment of 102 birth centers by the National Association of Childbearing Centers in 1983 showed 2.5 deaths per 1,000 births. Authors of the 1989 study attributed the improvement to better safety as a result of more widespread accreditation, self-scrutiny, and continuing education.

Chapter Ten

1. W. Schramm, D. Barnes, J. Bakewell, "Neonatal Mortality in Missouri Home Births, 1978–84," *American Journal of Public Health* 77 (8) (1987):930–935.

2. Ibid.
3. R. Anderson, D. Greener, "A Descriptive Analysis of Home Births Attended by CNMs in Two Nurse-Midwifery Services," *Journal of Nurse-Midwifery* 36 (2) (1991):95–103.
4. L. Alber, V. Katz, "Birth Setting for Low-Risk Pregnancies, An Analysis of the Current Literature," *Journal of Nurse-Midwifery* 36 (4) (1991):215–220.
5. Anderson et al., ibid.
6. Ibid.

Chapter Eleven
1. *The Cost of Maternity Care and Childbirth in the United States, 1989.* Research Bulletin R1589. Health Insurance Association of America, Washington, D.C., p. 8. Information provided by the National Association of Childbearing Centers.
2. F. Patch, and S. Holaday, "Effects of changes in professional liability insurance on certified nurse-midwives." *Journal of Nurse-Midwifery* 34 (3) (1989):131–136.
3. P. Langton, and D. Kammerer, "Childbearing and women's choice of nurse-midwives in Washington, D.C., hospitals." *Women & Health* 15 (2) (1989):49–65.
4. Report of the New York State Department of Health, Ad Hoc Advisory Committee on the Education and Recruitment of Midwives, June 1988, 5.
5. Ibid., 11.

Select Bibliography

Bean, Constance A. *Methods of Childbirth,* rev. ed. New York: William Morrow, 1990.

Crichton, Jennifer. *Delivery, A Nurse-Midwife's Story.* New York: Warner Books, 1986.

Ehrenreich, Barbara, and Deirdre English. *Witches, Midwives, and Nurses: A History of Women Healers.* New York: The Feminist Press at The City University of New York, 1973.

Eisenberg, A., H. Murkoff, and S. Hathway. *What to Expect When You're Expecting.* New York: Workman Publishing, 1984, 1988.

Hales, Dianne, and Timothy R.B. Johnson. *Intensive Caring, New Hope for High-Risk Pregnancy.* New York: Crown, 1990.

Hotchner, Tracy. *Pregnancy & Childbirth.* New York: Avon, 1979, 1984, 1990.

Kitzinger, Sheila. *Your Baby, Your Way.* New York: Pantheon, 1987.

Logan, Onnie Lee, as told to Katherine Clark. *Motherwit, An Alabama Midwife's Story.* New York: E.P. Dutton, 1989.

McCartney, Marion, CNM, and Antonia van der Meer. *The Midwife's Pregnancy & Childbirth Book.* New York: Henry Holt, 1990.

Ulrich, Laurel Thatcher. *A Midwife's Tale, The Life of Martha Ballard, Based on Her Diary, 1785–1812.* New York: Alfred A. Knopf, 1990.

Wertz, Richard W. and Dorothy C., *Lying-In, A History of Childbirth in America.* New York: The Free Press, 1977.

Index

THE AMERICAN COLLEGE OF NURSE MIDWIVES

The American College of Nurse Midwives, or ACNM, is the largest professional organization of midwives, representing four thousand certified nurse-midwives in the United States and abroad. ACNM regulates the education and certification of nurse-midwives, and it sets professional standards for their expert and compassionate approach to childbirth. Through a series of joint statements with the American College of Obstetricians and Gynecologists, nurse-midwives are acknowledged by the mainstream medical community as safe, capable caregivers for normal pregnancy and birth.

ABOUT THE AUTHOR

Sandra Jacobs is an editor for the Miami *Herald*. She is the former medical writer for the *Sun-Sentinel* newspaper in Fort Lauderdale. She has a master's degree in journalism from Columbia University and a bachelor's degree from Harvard College.